Chicken Soup for the Soul®
Healthy Living:
Stress

Chicken Soup for the Soul
Healthy Living:
Stress

Jack Canfield

Mark Victor Hansen

Leslie Godwin, MFCC

Health Communications, Inc.
Deerfield Beach, Florida

www.bcibooks.com
www.chickensoup.com

Library of Congress Cataloging-in-Publication Data
available from the Library of Congress

Publisher: Health Communications, Inc.
            3201 S.W. 15th Street
            Deerfield Beach, FL 33442-8190

Cover design by Larissa Hise Henoch
Inside book design by Lawna Patterson Oldfield
Inside book formatting by Dawn Von Strolley Grove

Contents

Fear less, hope more,
eat less, chew more,
whine less, breathe more,
talk less, say more,
love more,
and all good things
will be yours.

—Swedish Proverb

Introduction:
You Can Beat Stress

Are you feeling overwhelmed? Do you have physical symptoms that your doctor (or your instincts) tells you are stress-related? Or does a family member suffer from stress but hasn't yet taken steps to deal with it?

This book can help.

Stress is not a disease, but it can cause or exacerbate diseases. It's vague enough to be blamed for almost anything from a bad mood to a heart condition. Yet it's concrete enough to cause certain hormones to course through your bloodstream and affect your appetite, weight, skin, and even your heart and other vital organs.

Most of us would say we know what to do when we're stressed. Try to relax, maybe take a vacation or get a massage. But even if we follow through on these actions, are they the most effective ways we can spend the little time and energy left over in our busy lives? And are they simple and affordable so that we can make them part of our day-to-day routine? A vacation is a great way to temporarily relieve certain kinds of stress, but most of us can't afford to head out of town often enough to make a long-term difference. A biweekly massage might do the trick, but the costs add up quickly.

We've come up with simple, proven methods to beat stress and have given you a variety of these ideas to sample until you find the combination that works best for you. Start by taking the quiz on page 6 to identify your stress style. Then, fill out the brief worksheets or checklists in those sections that relate to your situation to see what you can do to reduce your stress right now. And enjoy the inspirational stories others have written and allowed us to share with you.

So don't forego the vacation you've been planning. And there's no need to cancel that massage you've scheduled. But read on to find out how you, or your loved ones, can reduce or eliminate stress by making simple changes in your attitude and behavior that will leave you feeling relaxed, energized and able to be fully engaged in your active life.

Take care.

—Leslie Godwin, MFCC, author of
From Burned Out to Fired Up

Looking for the Moon

"Moon, Mama," Jessica says, grabbing my arm and pointing at the window. She is obsessed with the moon. But until she was five years old, she didn't even know it existed. Before that, it was just the two of us and bright lights and hospital beds and a long and gradual awakening to awareness.

Once she discovered the moon and how it changes from one evening to the next, she fixated on it, demanding to know how it waxes and wanes. She memorized the words: "crescent" and "half," "gibbous" and "full." On her seventh birthday last July, the new moon had not yet risen. After she scanned the sky unsuccessfully, she asked with a sigh if I thought the dogs had eaten it.

I practice patience with her obsessions: rock collecting, the three songs we must sing in order before bed, Rudolph the Red-Nosed Reindeer and her shrill rejection of the word "little." Patience when she was a newborn and nobody could explain why she was having seizures; patience when she was seven months old and the neurologist finally gave a name to the illness—tuberous sclerosis, a rare disease that causes tumors and seizure disorder, and in Jessica's case, malformed her brain; patience when the surgeons removed most of the left side of her brain, leaving me to cope with the wreckage of my dreams and a little girl who couldn't even hold her head up. I know a lot about patience, more than I would like to know.

Sometimes my patience runs out, like right now, as I try to fix dinner while she demands that I look at the moon. She always stands precisely where I need to be next. It's little kid radar: how to best position herself where she cannot be ignored. In some regards, she is like every other child I have known.

I've got a heavy pan in one hand and a colander in the other, and I'm keeping an eye on the stove because the burner is still lit, and it would be just like Jessica to stick her hand on it. It doesn't matter how many times I tell her not to touch the stove, she doesn't remember. Her mind is like this colander. How many times have I told her? Ten thousand times. But then try to get her to forget something, like the word "dammit," or the phrase "your father is a pain in the ass."

"Moon, Mama!" Jessica says more urgently as I uncap the olive oil.

"Yes, the moon," I say absently. The phone rings.

I toss the drained noodles back in the pan, add a slosh of olive oil, wipe my hands on my jeans and answer the phone.

It's Publisher's Clearing House, but I know I'm not a winner and hang up. The oil sizzles on the stove, and I catch the pan up, narrowly avoiding a collision with Jessica.

"What kind of moon, Mama?" Jessica persists.

"I don't know. I can't see the moon," I say, tossing the noodles into a bowl. I wonder what happened to my wooden spoon. It was here a minute ago. And what did Jessica do with the Parmesan cheese? Jessica was probably trying to be helpful, and took it out of the refrigerator while I was on the phone, which would mean it's . . . where?

I look at the counter tops cluttered with dishes but don't see the cheese. I do find the spoon on the floor, just exactly where you'd expect it to be. I toss it into the sink, then scrabble through the drawers trying to find a substitute.

"What kind of moon, Mama?" Jessica raises her voice and plants herself in my path, thrusting her face toward mine. Sometimes she takes no prisoners.

"I don't know!" I say. "Where's the cheese? Where'd you put the damned cheese?"

Her eyes fill with tears. Great. How hard can it be to make spaghetti without causing your kid to cry? How hard can that be? I am sure other mothers accomplish it all the time.

I kneel down and take Jessica's face in my hands. "I'm sorry," I say. "I had a tough day today. And it's snowing again, and I'm tired, and I yelled when I shouldn't have."

The tears tremble for a moment.

"Can Mama have a big hug?" I ask, and I give her a big hug, and I say I love her and I'm sorry I yelled. I rock back on my heels and look into her big brown eyes. I want her to say it's okay, or that she's mad I yelled.

Instead, she looks up at me and says very seriously, "Moon is full."

Yes, indeed. Well, that's the main thing, I guess.

"The moon is full," I say, and ruffle my fingers through her short brown hair, and find the Parmesan cheese in the microwave, just where you'd expect it to be.

♥ *Jennifer Lawler*

Take a Deep Breath

You're on edge, jittery, anxious . . . you're *stressed*! Join the club. Between trying to cram more activities into less time, coping with life's challenges and taking care of loved ones, many of us are feeling the effects of stress.

Stress has plenty of negative effects on your body and mind. Ever get a tension headache? That's stress. Ever search frantically for the car keys—that you're holding in your hand? That can be stress, too. The good news is that if you regularly practice techniques to reduce stress, you'll reap such benefits as:

- Increased energy
- Better memory
- Enhanced ability to concentrate
- Greater patience and tolerance for typical frustrations

You don't have to spend your life in a scented bubble bath to stress less—you just have to make some healthy lifestyle changes. Let's get started! Take the "What's Your Stress Style?" quiz to learn the best way for *you* to de-stress.

WHAT'S YOUR STRESS STYLE?

1. When you're confronted by change or challenge, you:
   a) feel energized.
   b) want to put off dealing with it.
   c) feel that this is a normal part of life.
   d) worry about how it affects those you care about.
2. When you have several projects or activities happening within a short period of time, you:
   a) enjoy the busy pace.
   b) worry that you won't be able to cope.
   c) readily rise to the occasion.
   d) feel that as long as your loved ones are okay, you'll be okay.
3. You feel stressed when:
   a) you have too much down time.
   b) you have too much happening at once.
   c) you have too many responsibilities in which you can't control the outcome.
   d) your loved ones are sick or in crisis.

If you answered mostly As, you are Addicted to Adrenaline. You enjoy the adrenaline rush of a deadline or an intense project. You may not notice that the pace or the pressure are affecting you negatively.

What To Do: It's hard for you to tell when you're

stressed, so you'll need to make a conscious decision to lower your stress when your busy pace
affects your health, relationships, or ability to complete projects up to your standards.

**If you answered mostly Bs, you are Over-
whelmed.** You struggle with what others might
experience as a low level of stress. A meeting with
your boss, an unexpected visitor, or a sudden change
in plans can throw you for a loop.

What To Do: You've probably found it helpful to
have a routine you can count on. But when the unexpected happens, have a plan for how to get grounded
or centered again. For example, you can call a friend
who helps you feel calm, do a brief meditation session, use guided imagery, or work out.

**If you answered mostly Cs, you are Superman/
Superwoman.** You're not daunted by an ambitious
schedule or tense situation. But you tend to ignore
warning signs of stress and neglect your health and
well-being in the pursuit of your impressive goals.

What To Do: You would benefit from learning
early warning signs of stress—both physical and
emotional—such as noticing when your mind is
racing or when you feel rushed and impatient at
minor delays or frustrations. You'll also need to
make a conscious effort to slow your pace before
stress gets a foothold.

If you answered mostly Ds, you are a Caretaker. You tend to be more aware of the stress or suffering of those you care about than of your own needs. A sick child or a spouse struggling with a difficult boss is more likely to make you consciously aware of being stressed than your own illness or difficulties at work.

What To Do: It might help to realize that you can be more effective with others, or on the job, if you take good care of yourself. Just as flight attendants tell parents in the case of an emergency to put their own oxygen masks on before putting on their children's masks, you are better able to help your loved ones cope when you're calm, content and rested.

Think about . . .
why I want to de-stress

The reasons I want to de-stress are:

__ To increase my energy

__ To improve my memory

__ To improve my ability to concentrate

__ To do a better job at work

__ To enhance my sense of well-being

__ To improve my patience

Other: _____

_____

_____

The Invisible Thief

Over the years I experienced two major stress-related burnouts on the job. Co-workers may beg to disagree and add a few more, but I count two.

Early in my career the small start-up I worked for became an overnight success and grew rapidly. We added people quickly, and they were expected to hit the ground running. Computers were just being introduced to small businesses, promising to be the solution to all our problems—eventually. I grappled with issues in a competitive industry I knew very little about and in my spare time searched for the secrets to managing different personalities and skill levels. In learning on the job through trial and error, I discovered I was good with technology and tasks but less so with people. At least some of the job got covered; problem was, all of it needed to be.

I put my nose closer to the grindstone, worked harder and smarter, and absorbed all the stress the universe could throw at me like a badge of honor.

When I could no longer crawl out of the well of self-denial or keep my game face on every day, I cried "uncle." Thinking it was the root of the problem, I kicked a substance abuse problem and motored on. It took a few more years for the realization to hit that an addictive personality remains addictive; it just substitutes a different substance. In my sobriety, I ended up replacing the high with more adrenaline and stress.

When my second burnout occurred, I had twenty-plus years of stress I could claim as my own—most of it self-imposed. I lashed out, acted inappropriately, was defiant, resistant to change, impatient . . . the list read like a textbook, and I felt like a bomb waiting to explode. But like many type A personalities, much of that behavior was looked upon (or overlooked) favorably because I got results and was successful. On a daily basis, most emotions got internalized. Feelings were shared and vented only with a small group of trusted friends, a group that suffered from attrition and grew smaller each year. I began to dread sitting down at my desk. I couldn't remember the last time I'd felt challenged, interested or turned on by what I did for a living. Instead I felt tired, unhappy, unappreciated, ineffective, negative, overwhelmed and depressed.

My home and husband were my refuge, but the cumulative effect of work-related stress was detrimental to my physical, spiritual and emotional well-being. I gained weight, felt fatigued, developed a chronic illness and had no desire to do anything but come home and trance-out in front of the television until my mind went numb.

Thankfully, the new millennium had dawned and was shining a spotlight on a kinder, gentler workplace. A balanced lifestyle, identifying problems and taking responsibility for the changes in one's life to nurture well-being, not a job or ideal, was becoming culturally acceptable. I was a co-conspirator undermining my well-being, aiding and abetting an invisible thief stealing small pieces of my tranquility on a regular basis until I was running on empty. I saw the light. I didn't need to wait for a career crisis or a life-threatening health issue to hit me over the head—I was close enough to the edge to know it was there.

I joined the gym—and went. I began to meditate—daily. I looked at my life and took an honest inventory of where I was and what I wanted. I prioritized the things that I got the most pleasure from and started to fill my day with those activities, people and ideas. Gradually my tolerance for dysfunction diminished, replaced by my desire to be surrounded by healthy, positive things and people. I took small steps and made gradual, determined changes, always mindful not to put more stress on myself in the process of learning to reduce it.

Slowly but surely I began to feel better. My perspective shifted and I began to redefine myself. I recognized that I was consumed by the addictive insidiousness of stress; its physiological effect on my body and my psyche, the adrenaline rush that kept the veil of depression at bay, and the excuse it gave me for not taking responsibility for myself and being more available to my family and friends.

A period of reorganization at work gave me the opportunity to make a significant change in my responsibilities, and I took it eagerly. We tightened the budget and made some lifestyle adjustments. It didn't take long to realize the benefit outweighed the risk. I got reacquainted with feeling challenged, learning new skills, exploring my spirit, discovering my creativity and living life rather than watching it.

Today I am healthy, and I feel strong, balanced and well—a thousand times better than I did at twenty-five when I began my long waltz with stress. People who have a basis for comparison say I look better as well. I see abundance every day and have never been happier in my work.

When that lightbulb went off a couple of years ago, I didn't know what to expect. What I discovered was a new paradigm—positive stress! I still thrive on hard work, challenges and that rush of adrenaline when a deadline looms, but my body, mind and spirit are healthy enough to appreciate the experience and reap the rewards. I intend to keep it that way.

♥ *Mary Reginald*

Stress and Your Health

Ever wonder why you keep catching colds? Stress may be the culprit, because it suppresses your immune system. And that's not all. Stress can cause frequent headaches, stomach distress, depression, dyshydrotic eczema (itchy, prickly blisters, usually on the hands), and even more serious problems—like a heart attack. According to one recent study, working under deadlines can trigger a heart attack, and an intense deadline can increase your risk six times, especially in the first twenty-four hours after the deadline.

The stress hormone adrenaline raises blood pressure and may even cause high blood sugar. It also increases the chances of cardiovascular disease, which could lead to a heart attack or stroke.

Stress can also make you fat. That's because of the stress hormone cortisol, which causes you to crave comfort foods like chocolate chip cookies and mashed potatoes. How many times have you found yourself digging into a pint of ice cream when you're feeling rushed or stressed?

Don't feel discouraged! In later sections, we'll tell you how to beat stress—and boost your health—through diet, exercise and other means.

Stress and Your Mood

Stress can make even the most cheerful person moody, irritable and quick to snap at those they love most. After a while, this can cause serious damage to those relationships.

IS STRESS AFFECTING YOUR MOOD?

The answer may be yes if you often feel:

__ Moody, sad, or withdrawn

__ Serious and no fun to be around

__ Irritable and impatient

__ Controlling

__ Distracted and not "in the moment"

__ Overly focused on the needs of others

__ Like you need a drink to relax

TIPS FOR BEATING THE MOODY BLUES

• If people close to you tell you that you've been moody or difficult to be with, try not to get defensive. Instead, ask for an example, or ask them to point out the behavior they're concerned about when it's happening. Then consider whether they have a point.

• If they have a point, thank them for letting you know and tell them you'll work on it.

• Work on your part of the problem even if

others are contributing to your reaction. Once you've changed your behavior, you can reevaluate the relationship. Others may even be more willing to look at their roles in the problem once they see that you're making a sincere effort.

Stress and Alcohol (and Drug) Abuse

A drink at the end of a long, difficult day is a part of our culture. But relying on alcohol or drugs to relax on a regular basis can cause problems. In fact, stress can affect how quickly your body absorbs alcohol, making that drink even more potent!

Quiz:

1. Do you ever feel you should cut back on your drinking or drug use?
2. Do others complain about your drinking or drug use?
3. Do you ever feel guilty after using drugs or alcohol? Do you ever regret your behavior while you were under the influence?
4. Does your drinking or drug use ever get in the way of your family responsibilities, job, or other relationships or obligations?

If you answered yes to any of these questions, please see your doctor.

☼ Think about . . .
what stress is doing to me

__ I often feel irritable and moody.

__ My friends and family say I can be difficult to be around.

__ I often have a drink to "take the edge off."

__ I get frequent colds.

__ I find myself craving comfort foods after a bad day.

__ I have high blood pressure.

__ I have a skin disorder that my doctor says is stress-related.

__ I often forget names and where I put things.

Other: _____

_____

_____

I'm experiencing these symptoms:

__ Chest pains

__ Trouble sleeping

__ Changes in my appetite or weight

__ Anxiety, irritability, sadness, a "dead" feeling or lack of enjoyment of things I usually enjoy

__ Exhaustion, frequent illness, feeling rundown much of the time

__ Stomach upset, cramping, diarrhea or constipation

__ Headaches, migraines, jaw pain, back or neck aches or spasms

__ Worsening of an ongoing condition, including skin conditions

Smell the Flowers

My friend Anita is the CEO of an export-import company. She is a well-heeled, high-flying, top-of-the-rung professional. She is also a hung-up, stressed-out, willing-to-climb-walls-and-tear-her-hair-out kind of person.

Anita has tried to find solutions for stress. She has a punching bag hidden in one of her office closets. Her top drawer has a couple of dolls that she can prick with colored pins. In her purse, she carries an aromatherapy bottle complete with inhaler, to breathe in positive feelings and breathe out negative ones.

Yet, she suffers, finding that these are not what the doctor ordered. Even what the doctor has ordered does not help because medication provides only short-term solutions. She is a victim, like most of us, of the mad rush that embodies life in the twenty-first century.

There is no limit to the way we stretch ourselves. We consider ourselves demigods and continuously tap on our resources to do that extra job, meet another deadline. Our shoulders droop, our eyes close, our mind boggles, but we carry on. "Ours is not to question why, ours is but to do and die," is the war cry or modern-day mantra of the super-self. What we fail to realize is that we are not at war with the world. Nor do we have to soldier on relentlessly. Our bodies need time to replenish and recoup, or we will falter and fall. All our achievements will come to naught if we do not have the time and energy to appreciate and enjoy them.

Stress is the way our body reacts to our attempts to overachieve. It is a scream for help. Continuous stress leads to hypertension, heart disease, ulcers, diabetes or psychological breakdown. That is why the incidence of such ailments is increasing every day. We have learned how to reach for the sky, but we haven't learned how to enjoy stars that twinkle there. We need time to rediscover ourselves, to rejuvenate our spirit, to reflect on the beauty of the world around us.

I cajoled Anita into attending a series of lectures with me. These centered on the long-term effects of stress, what causes it and how we can try to de-stress ourselves. One of the stories we heard was how a very successful man walked to his office in a high-rise building every day. He walked, despite owning a fleet of cars, because he was a health-conscious, modern-day businessman. It irked him (stressed him!) to see a man sitting by the riverside each day, whiling away his time fishing. One day, despite his structured schedule, he strolled up to the fisherman and asked him if he knew the value of time, work and money. He said that if the man did some sensible work in the time he spent fishing, he could earn a lot of money. The fisherman looked up and asked what that would help him achieve. The businessmen said that he could then sit back and relax.

"What do you think I'm doing now?" was the fisherman's rejoinder. He then turned back to his fishing, his face peaceful. The businessman walked on, his mind in chaos. The next day there were two men fishing without a care in the world.

Anita has decided to make some changes in her lifestyle in order to become more relaxed. She has cut back on a busy schedule and meets her parents every weekend in the country. Here she unwinds in their gentle company and reads a book, takes a walk with the dogs or listens to music. She rolls on the grass and smells the flowers. When she returns to the glass and steel structure of her office on Mondays, she is refreshed and exhilarated, ready to take on the world.

She tells me that she has thrown the voodoo dolls into the wastebasket, uses the punching bag as a footrest and the aroma inhalant as a room purifier.

♥ *Abha Iyengar*

Returning to the Sunlight

Some of the worst stress I ever experienced was at my first engineering job, fresh out of graduate school. I had the bad luck to start my career in Silicon Valley at the very start of the tech crash; it was all downhill from the day I started.

Our department was a very close-knit and friendly group of about ten people. Most of them had worked together for years; some had been with the company for as long as twenty-five years. It was originally a very pleasant place to work: people would chat and joke with each other, one could always count on one's co-workers to answer questions or to help, and the managers were very friendly with the people they managed.

A year after I started my job, the layoffs began. The management never told us who was being laid off next; almost every Tuesday we had a surprise. Obviously, this wreaked havoc with everyone's nerves. My once-friendly boss started avoiding people and snarling at everyone who came near his cubicle. Some of my co-workers lost their motivation and stopped working altogether. Some tried to sabotage their co-workers. Others tried to hold things together, working fourteen-hour days in an effort to get everything done. When people got pink slips, everyone else avoided them; they'd pack up their stuff in silence and depart quietly, as if they were invisible. The only topic of conversation was the next layoff: when it would be, who'd be laid off, what higher management was thinking.

I felt the stress just like everyone else. I worked a lot; I'd go to work before the sun rose and come home when it was already dark. I had trouble sleeping, I had wild mood swings, and when I was at work I wanted to cry all the time. But I kept telling myself that it was worth it, it was what jobs were like, and what other choice was there?

I got laid off after working too many fourteen-hour days in a row. I'd spent so long dreading that moment that it came as a relief when it finally happened. I started frantically looking for a new job. The job hunting was just as intense, and just as stressful, as the job I left. I went to job counseling, worked and worked on my resume, attended networking groups, donned my formal suit for interviews. I kept in touch with my former co-workers, and knew that things weren't getting better at my former workplace.

And then came the funerals. Some of my former

co-workers weren't all that young, or all that healthy, and the stress got to them. One died of a heart attack shortly after getting laid off. He'd been with the company twenty-four years. Another one died of a perforated ulcer at a relatively young age.

I attended both of the funerals. The second one was particularly painful. It was hard to look at the raw grief that showed in the faces of the man's wife and teenage sons, hard to listen to all the eulogies and to think about the life cut short—by work? For the greater glory of the corporation? When did work become so important that we are now expected to sacrifice our lives to it?

I walked out of the funeral home and decided to skip the job-hunting meeting I had that day. Instead, I went to the park near my house; it had a gorgeous trail winding through the pine forest. I walked the trail slowly, looking up at the sun, and suddenly realized that I hadn't felt the sun on my face for at least a year. I'd never been outside during the day; I was always indoors working.

When I came back from the park, I went straight to Kinko's and printed up colorful flyers advertising myself as a piano teacher, math tutor, translator, accompanist—everything I could think of. The very next day, I had my first client. Within three weeks, I was self-supporting.

I've been happily self-employed for two years

now. I set my own hours, determine my own work-
load. I am finally in control of my own life. I work
just as hard, but without the constant stress hanging over my head, without the worries of what my
boss or higher management would think. And
every day, I take a walk outside and feel the warm
sunshine on my face.

♥ *Larisa Migachyov*

On-the-Job Stress

Your co-worker is snapping her gum (again), and the boss wants that report done—yesterday. Meanwhile, you're frantically getting ready for yet another business trip. The workplace is a typical, but challenging, source of stress. How stressful is your job? Check the statements below that are true for you:

SEVERE STRESSORS

___ My boss has unrealistic expectations of me/my team.

___ I'm expected to work up to a standard I wasn't trained to meet.

___ I have a lot of responsibility but little control over getting projects done the way I believe they should be done.

___ I travel a lot on business (and do not enjoy it).

___ There have been layoffs, a merger or a buyout at my company within the last year.

___ I work with one or two difficult people, including my boss.

MODERATE STRESSORS

___ My boss is pleasant but just not around very much when I need help.

___ I am qualified to do my job, but because of

layoffs or budget problems, I have more work to do than can realistically get done each day.

__ I have a lot of responsibility, but most of the time I have the authority to get projects done the way I believe they should be done.

__ I travel a lot on business (which I enjoy).

__ I work with one or two difficult people, not including my boss.

How did you fare? One or more *severe* stressors can make your worklife very difficult and can cause you to bring work stress home from the office. This isn't only frustrating for you, it can have a powerful impact on your family. A new study showed that men with wives who come home stressed from work are more than twice as likely to develop heart disease than those without such stress.

One *moderate* stressor is tolerable (and typical) in most workplaces. Depending on your sensitivity to stress, it could cause chronic mild symptoms like irritability or moderate overeating. But more than one moderate stressor at the same time, for example, frequent travel that you enjoy plus working with a difficult person other than your boss, can cause more severe symptoms.

WHAT TO DO AT WORK

- Try to separate what pushes your buttons in your work environment from what is objectively stressful.

- Bring up the objective stressors with your boss to get help solving the problem. For example, if you're expected to use a new computer program to develop a report, but you haven't been trained to use the program, ask for a training session or for the vendor to come in to teach you how to do the job.

- When you treat problems as *business* problems, you and your boss are on the same side. If you treat them as personal attacks, you'll either expect your boss to rescue you, or you'll feel that he or she isn't being supportive.

- If you're stressed because you prefer to be in control of all aspects of a project, but you're expected to work as part of a team, this might not be the fault of your workplace. Your job might not be a good match for your personality. Either consider a different job, or decide that you'd like to get used to working as a member of a team and limiting your control to your own contribution.

WHAT TO DO OUTSIDE OF WORK

- Pay attention to whether you're bringing your stress home from work. Everyone has a bad day once in a while, but do any of these describe how you are on a regular basis at home?
  - __ irritable
  - __ impatient
  - __ disappointed that your kids and spouse don't do chores the way you want them done
  - __ quick to become angry or frustrated
  - __ blue on Sunday evenings at the thought of going back to work
- Pay attention to your interactions with your children and spouse. Do you treat them like they're the most important people in your life? If not, how can you let them know by your actions and attitude that you love and cherish them?
- If you've changed your behavior but you still need to talk to your children or spouse about their behavior and how it upsets you, choose a calm moment and talk about one thing that you believe they do that is unpleasant or rude. Don't give them a laundry list, and be willing to hear their side of the story.
- Do something on your way home to transition from employee or boss to mom or dad or

husband or wife. Change your clothes, stop at the gym, listen to uplifting music on the ride home, or simply drive in silence, quiet your mind and let all your work thoughts go. When you cross the threshold of your home, consciously decide to be in the moment and enjoy your family or alone time.

• Work on the suggestions presented in this book to lower your stress level.

It's natural to bring work stress home. But once you get in the habit of reducing your stress at work, you'll feel a lot more relaxed when it's time to go home and greet your family!

Think about . . .
my work stress

What stresses me out about work?

_____

_____

_____

Do I bring my work stress home?

_____

_____

_____

Can I bring up the work stressors with my boss?

_____

_____

_____

If so, here's what I'll say to my boss, so I sound
proactive instead of complaining:

_____

_____

_____

Am I willing to talk to my family about how they can support my decision to make some changes?

_____

_____

_____

Here's what I'll say to my family so they can support me:

_____

_____

_____

My Mother's Strength

When I was just fourteen, I watched my mother age ten years in a sickly green hospital room. It was cancer, and I knew it was bad because although I had seen my mother bear many crosses in her life, I had never seen her face look so drawn, tired and hopeless.

For my mother, though, this cancer was more than another cross to bear. She believed she was watching me, her youngest daughter, die.

Through the glass walls of my hospital room I could see the doctor and my mother. As the young resident started talking, my mother's head fell back and tears started streaming down her face. Her arms flailed in despair.

When she walked into my hospital room with the doctor, she looked like she had just been dealt the knockout blow of her life. Her eyes stared pleadingly at the doctor. She wanted me to know— I had that right—but she just couldn't be the one to tell me.

And when the doctor sat on the side of the bed

and put his cold, clammy hand on my arm, I knew I was really, really sick. But it was when I looked over at my mother's face—which had gone from a youthful, smiling one with dancing eyes to the haggard, lackluster one before me—that I knew I was dying.

It was Hodgkin's disease. My fourteen-year-old body was riddled with cancerous tumors. The doctor sugar-coated nothing. He told me of the incredible pain I would endure. He told me of the weight I would lose and all the hair that would fall out. The doctors would try to shrink the existing tumors with chemotherapy and radiation therapy, but that was no guarantee. There was the very good chance that I would never turn fifteen.

My head fell back on the pillow, and I closed my eyes. I wanted to shut it all out and run away. When the doctor left the room, I wanted to believe that all the ugliness was walking out the door with him. *Maybe,* I thought, *when I opened my eyes, my mother's face would look young again, and we could go home and bake one of my infamous lopsided cakes.*

Instead, when I opened my eyes, my mother, sitting beside me, took my hand, pursed her lips and said determinedly, "We'll get through this."

During my stay at the hospital, my mother arrived in my room every morning and stayed there until the last seconds of the last visiting hour at night. For most of the day no words passed between us except for the occasional, "Pat, you should eat something." I spent my days staring out of the window while my mother sat and read or watched television. There was absolutely no pressure to talk about the situation. It wasn't profound words of support and love that entwined our souls. It was simply my mother letting me be.

Three weeks later, on the morning I was to be released from the hospital, my mother brought me my favorite bell-bottom jeans, tie-dyed blouse and Earth shoes. Seeing them perked me up like no medication in that entire hospital could. I couldn't wait to wear them.

My mother drew the curtains, and I, like any other clothes-crazy teenager, dressed with great glee. When I pulled up the jeans and buttoned them, I could tell right away that they were not mine. They couldn't be, because they fell off the once rounded hips they used to hug so nicely. I was incredulous. In the hospital gown I hadn't noticed the ravages of illness.

I yelled at my mother as though it was her fault. "You brought the wrong jeans! These are too big!" I screamed.

My mother just walked out of the room and went out to the nurse's station, returning immediately with two safety pins. "Look," she said, "it will be all right. All we have to do is pin them up here in the back. Your top will cover them."

"No, I don't want to pin them. I want them to fit right," I sulked, and folding my arms, sat on the bed and cried to the wall.

When I finally looked over at my mother, her eyes boring into mine, I realized that I had to pin my pants. Without saying a word, she was telling me: No matter how much you pout, cry and stomp like a mule, these pants are not going to fit right without these pins. You are sick. Your body is not the same. You have to accept this.

It was then that I learned to compromise with my mother, and with a force larger than myself—a force I could not see, or hear, or touch, but a force that nonetheless had taken control of my life.

Though I left the hospital knowing the doctors believed that I would only return to die, none of it ever felt completely real. My body was disintegrating, I could barely walk and I couldn't keep food down, but death felt as far away from me as grandmotherhood. I don't know why I had this feeling. Maybe it was because my fourteen-year-old mind couldn't grasp the concept of mortality, or perhaps I felt something telling me that this wasn't going to be the end.

I quickly slipped into the normalness of everyday life at home, surrounded by my mother and my sisters. And my mother and I, in the face of my illness, discovered a special way of being together.

We knew what was destroying my body, but we never said the words *cancer* or *death*. Still, on a day when I was too weak even to feed myself, I looked up at my mother as she was feeding me some mashed food, and something in me felt that one, if not both, of those words needed to be spoken.

"Mommy," I finally said after about the third swallow, "am I really going to die?"

My mother dropped the bowl of food, spilling it all over me and broke into uncontrollable tears that would not stop, no matter how hard I pleaded with her.

I was frozen with fear. I couldn't take back what I had said. Besides, I really wanted to know. If my mother would just confirm it one way or another, whatever she said would be what was real.

Finally, she looked up at me and said, "My baby is not going to die. Do you hear me? I don't ever want to hear you say that again. Do you hear me?"

I heard her. I never said it again. I simply went about the business of fighting for my life.

Yet as my body withered to eighty-two pounds and my hair fell out, I could see how helpless my mother felt. Her hair grew grayer. She even matched me, pound for pound, with the weight she lost. And yet, it was her strength that jump-started my will to make my frail body walk instead of ride in a wheel-chair. It was her strength that helped me walk into school wearing a wig amidst stares and whispers from pretty, healthy-bodied girls. And it was her strength that made me see that in the larger picture, those stares and whispers didn't mean a thing.

More than a year went by before I finally went into remission. When the doctor called my mother and me into his office after the last chemotherapy treatment, we didn't know what to expect. Somehow, though, we knew we didn't need to expect the worst. He went through a long-winded dissertation about shrunken tumors and good cell counts before he told us, essentially, that I was in remission.

My mother and I didn't cry tears of joy. We didn't get swept up in a whirl of happiness and gid-diness, hugging the stuffing out of each other. We just smiled and squeezed each other's hands. The doctor was really only telling us something that we already knew: that I was not going to die.

♥ *Patricia Jones*

When Someone
You Love Is Stressed

SPOUSE STRESS

Your spouse has become irritable, forgetful and moody. It's stress! It can be nerve-racking to live with, and love, a stressed-out spouse or partner. You probably know from experience that it's not always easy to tell when *you're* stressed. In the same way, your loved one may not realize when *he or she* is suffering from stress. So what can you do? Try these tips:

- Ask your loved one to take the quiz on page 6.
- Be empathic, but don't make excuses for him or her.
- Point out how your loved one's stress is affecting you, the kids, or his or her work as objectively as you can.
- Don't allow a stressed out spouse to be rude. If he or she is verbally or physically abusive, get professional or legal help.
- Don't complain about how your loved one is stressing you out. Take responsibility for your stress while offering support and trying to understand what he or she going through.

KID STRESS

Childhood should be a time of play and learning—a carefree and happy time before having to face adult responsibilities and worries.

But for many children, childhood is a difficult time where they're bombarded by stressors with causes beyond their control. A Kids Health° Kids Poll survey of 1,004 nine- to thirteen-year-olds shows that 20 to 30 percent of these children worried daily. Topping the list of worries were those about their appearance (43 percent), problems at home (39 percent), and being liked (33 percent). They also worried about being a failure or disappointing their loved ones (29 percent), and they worried about their friends and their friends' problems (27 percent).

STRESS AND YOUR YOUNG CHILD

Young children are stressed when their needs aren't being met appropriately and consistently. Their dependence on their parents or other primary caregivers means they'll feel stress when these relationships change.

You should be concerned if your young child:

__ Shows changes in typical behavior like crying, eating, sleeping or fussiness without a physical cause

___ Becomes more clingy
___ Becomes less affectionate
___ Becomes more angry or more likely to have tantrums
___ Gives you any other reason to believe that something is wrong

WORKSHEET FOR PARENTS OF YOUNG CHILDREN

1. What behavior shows that your child is stressed? (Use the checklist above.)
2. Are there changes in your child's routine or stressors at home? What are they?
3. What can you do to reassure your child or prevent the stressor?
   ___ Read her a book about the stressful situation, such as *Berenstain Bears Go to the Dentist* or *The Fall of Freddie the Leaf* (which is about death and loss).
   ___ Explain in simple terms what is happening or going to happen.
   ___ Help your child express her feelings in words and by drawing pictures.

STRESS AND YOUR SCHOOL-AGED CHILD

School-aged children are still susceptible to the stressors of losses or other changes at home, but are also becoming wrapped up in the outside world of friends, school and after-school activities. These relationships have a lot of influence over your child's sense of well-being.

You should be concerned if your child:

__ Begins bed-wetting

__ Has frequent stomachaches

__ Has trouble sleeping or is sleeping much more than usual

__ Bullies other children or is bullied himself

__ Frequently disobeys or shows anger

__ Is withdrawn or depressed

__ Tries to tune out through excessive TV watching or video game playing

WORKSHEET FOR PARENTS OF SCHOOL-AGED CHILDREN

1. What behavior shows that your child is stressed? (Use the checklist above.)
2. Are there changes in your child's routine or stressors at home? What are they?
3. Is there a bully at school? If so, talk to that child's parents and the principal or adults in charge.
4. What else can you do?
   __ Explain what to expect.
   __ Help your child express his feelings in words; journal with your child.
   __ Be very clear about your expectations for

your child. Unclear expectations can be stressful. For example, if you've always taught her that you care most about her character, don't put more emphasis on her grades than what kind of person she is.

STRESS AND YOUR TEEN

From raging hormones to more responsibility, teens have many reasons to be stressed. And it's hard for parents to figure out if their teen is moody because he's a normal, hormonal teen, or if there's a more serious problem that needs parental support or intervention. Stakes are now higher for both parents and teens. A troubled teen with access to alcohol and a car is capable of serious damage to himself and others. On the other hand, a parent who overreacts to a teen's normal moodiness could hamper the communication that's essential to preventing serious problems.

You should be concerned if your teen:

__ Has mood swings
__ Appears high or drunk
__ Is frequently ill
__ Is sad, very tired, or unhappy much of the time
__ Has more energy and needs less sleep than usual

__ Has sudden changes in friends, grades or behavior

__ Is defensive much of the time

__ Tries to tune out through excessive TV watching or video game playing

WORKSHEET FOR PARENTS OF TEENS

1. What behavior shows that your teen is stressed? (Use the checklist above.)

2. What has changed recently in his or her routine or life?

3. What stressors does your teen have? Has anything changed in these areas?
   __ friendships, romantic relationships
   __ at school, preparation for college or work
   __ learning to drive
   __ graduating high school

4. What can you do?
   __ Spend more "down" time together to encourage communication and connection.
   __ Be more curious about his or her interests.
   __ Get more involved in his or her school or extracurricular activities.
   __ Know who his or her friends (and friends' parents) are.
   __ Get him or her a professional consultation or evaluation.
   __ Have your teen take a drug test.

Time to Play

The phone was about to ring. My deadline was looming. Meanwhile, my daughters were whiny and irascible, both on the brink of a meltdown as they burrowed themselves in surly, uncompromising moods. It was a late weekday afternoon, and my two worlds—that of freelance writer and stay-at-home mother—were about to collide in one ugly showdown.

It was I who created this disaster, which was now my life. Before giving birth, I'd been a newspaper reporter. I quit to do what I believed was the noble thing and became a full-time, stay-at-home mom. I lasted only two months on the job before I began looking for something else.

What I didn't realize was how much I would miss the thrill of working and spending my days with smart, intriguing people who didn't need me to burp them. To make matters worse, it was winter, and I was recovering from a C-section while trapped in a tiny apartment with a baby who had nightly crying jags, then refused to sleep more than two hours at a time. I knew my mental state was precarious when I started looking forward to *Colombo* reruns.

So two months after Samantha was born, I decided to become a freelance magazine writer. I'd done some freelance work in the past. I liked the flexibility and freedom that freelancing promised and reveled in the challenge of landing an assignment. I also liked finding a check in the mail and the thrill of seeing my name in a national magazine.

Freelancing while trying to raise kids, however, was an entirely different ballgame. At first, it didn't seem so bad. The work was slow, and I kept my ambitions in check. When I did land an assignment or two, I worked during Samantha's naps. But as I started getting more ambitious and the work started coming in, life got increasingly insane, especially after the birth of my second daughter, Stephanie. Only hours after coming home from the hospital with her, I was on e-mail answering an editor's questions.

Part of the problem was that I resisted hiring babysitting. I didn't make enough to justify hiring a full-time sitter. I also believed it was my duty to raise my kids, and I loved being there for all their precious moments and milestones. So with the exception of a weekly visit from my mother and some occasional help from my mother-in-law, I had little outside assistance. Instead, I worked in the evenings and on the weekends, when my husband was home and could tend to my daughters.

But as any writer knows, you can't control when a source will return your calls or when an editor will be on the phone looking for that last shred of information. To get my work done, I relied heavily on e-mail and frequently looked for sources in California who were three hours behind me. I also tried to make appointments for phone interviews that coincided with nap time.

Even so, there were days like this one, when everything had slipped out of my control, and I was left with unpredictability. Why couldn't the source have called when Stephanie was napping? What will I do if one of the girls starts beckoning for my attention while I'm on the phone? What if they start fighting and shouting at the tops of their lungs? How was I going to conduct a coherent interview with a source who assumed I was a professional writer, not a mother with frazzled nerves on the verge of a breakdown?

I looked at the mess that had become our family room, and it suddenly dawned on me that there was little I could do to stop my kids from throwing a wicked tantrum and even less I could do to make the phone ring. After all, I couldn't control what other people did or how they felt. I certainly wasn't in charge of anyone's schedule, much less that of a stranger. But I was in charge of me, and the only thing that really mattered was what was happening now, at this moment.

So I took a deep breath and sat down in the middle of all the Legos, stuffed animals and Barbie dolls. "Come here girls," I told my daughters. They stopped what they were doing and walked into my embrace. I held them close in tight, delicious hugs that I wished could last forever. In a single instant, I felt better about everything. We played, and I let myself get lost in building a Lego house. The source didn't call until the next day. By then, everyone was in a happier mood.

♥ *Winnie Yu*

The Serenity Prayer

God, grant me the serenity to accept
the things I cannot change,
The courage to change the things I can,
And the wisdom to know the difference.

Mission Control

Though the origin of "The Serenity Prayer" is unknown, it's been used by Alcoholics Anonymous and other 12-step programs since 1942. "The Serenity Prayer" has helped countless alcoholics and addicts, as well as their loved ones. It's a beautifully simple way to ask for guidance, or simply to remember that there are many aspects of life that we care about deeply but cannot control.

Even though most of us have heard "The Serenity Prayer" before, few of us have really stopped to consider what it means.

- Having the *serenity to accept what we can't change* doesn't mean we're happy with the outcome. It does mean that we've made peace with what was inevitable.
- Having the *courage to change the things we can* doesn't mean we automatically know exactly what to do or feel good about doing it. It means that we're willing to figure out how to handle something difficult because that's the right thing to do.
- Having the *wisdom to know the difference*—that is the real crux of this prayer. Until we know what we can and can't control, we're stuck trying to control other people or circumstances

over which we have no authority. Or we avoid taking action because we don't realize that we can make a difference.

- Asking for *clarity* is critical to understanding our role in the world—one moment, one action and one intention at a time.

Think about . . .
can I control this stress?

What am I stressed about right now?
(For example, "I don't have enough money to
pay my child's tuition this month.")

_____

_____

_____

_____

What about this stressor is out of my control? It
may be that it is under someone else's control
or simply is not controllable.
(For example, "My ex-husband is behind on
child support payments. I can't control his
willingness to pay, his income or his ability
to make payments.")

_____

_____

_____

_____

What about this stressor can I control? This may be my reaction, or it can include concrete steps I can take.

(For example, "I can contact my lawyer to see how to enforce the payment schedule decreed by the judge; I can talk to the financial aid department at my child's school to see if there are scholarships or other options; I can practice letting go of the stress once I've identified there's nothing more I can do.")

_____

_____

_____

_____

Kicking Stress

My typical day goes something like this:

9:00 A.M. Wake up, drive to work, drink coffee.

1:00 P.M. First meal of the day: frozen micro-wave meal.

3:00 P.M. Second meal of the day: peanut-butter M&Ms and Gummi Bears.

4:00 P.M. Second cup of coffee (vital).

6:00 P.M. Drive home.

6:30 P.M. Collapse on couch. Think about cooking. Realize there's nothing to cook and no way of cooking it. Eat take-out, fast food or second frozen dinner.

7:00 P.M. Glass of wine while watching television.

10:00 P.M. Sleep, fitfully.

9:00 A.M. Repeat.

I'm twenty-two years old, and I'm exhausted. Walking up a flight of stairs makes my heart pound. I grind my teeth every night. I have no energy, and I don't know how to get it back.

I've just graduated from college in New York and moved across the country to Los Angeles. In the home of the tanned and the toned, I am neither. In the past four years, my only exercise consisted of raising my arm to feed myself macaroni and cheese.

It wasn't always this way. In junior high and high school, I was extremely active, partially because the Illinois Department of Education requires students to take an hour of gym each day.

The summer before college, I even indulged my fantasy of becoming a ninja by signing up for tae kwon do (the Korean form of karate). An obvious goal was to earn my black belt, but secretly my favorite color belt was light blue. It was by far the prettiest shade, and I longed to tie it around my uniform, called a *dobuk*. Though I loved every second of class, I never followed up with the exercises while at college. By my sophomore year, I gave up on ninja-hood completely.

Several years passed before fate smacked me upside the head. My apartment in L.A. was a mere block from a reputable martial arts school. One morning before work, I gingerly walked inside the dojang to pick up a brochure and class schedule. I glanced at the wall where the belts hung and mentally catalogued them: white, yellow, orange, purple, green, dark blue, red, red with stripe, brown, brown with stripe and black. *Hmmm. Where was light blue?*

The trial lesson that night left me aching from head to toe. The following morning I could barely move.

It felt great.

On the second day, I blacked out halfway through class. I wasn't hurt, just really humiliated. Grandmaster Jin Hwan Kim sternly advised me to change my eating and drinking habits. Specifically, he told me to always eat breakfast and drink at least eight glasses of water on the days I had class.

Pride would never let me publicly collapse again, so I began eating cereal or oatmeal for breakfast on Mondays, Wednesdays and Fridays. Soon my stomach growled so loudly when I woke up that I decided to feed it every morning.

Because it was considered horribly rude to show up in a wrinkled or unclean uniform, laundry took on a frequency it had never previously known. I still didn't cook much, but I had energy now and felt my arms and legs growing stronger every week. The intense workouts delivered a burst of adrenaline that boosted my spirits and later helped me fall asleep at night.

Occasionally martial arts itself was a source of stress. Belt testing and sparring sessions made me nervous, but also taught me that I could overcome physical and mental challenges through practice and determination.

Now it's five years later, and I'm a first-degree black belt in tae kwon do and hapkido. The final test consisted of five hours of meditation, three days of fasting, several separate physical exams and countless credit hours teaching other students. Most important, earning my black belt helped me become healthy again. (Another positive side-effect: I learned that I do, in fact, have abs.)

It sure would have been nice to get that light blue belt, though. . . .

♥ *Sarah Skilton*

Beating Stress Eating

Trouble at work? Have a pint of Ben & Jerry's New York Super Fudge Chunk. Got a test coming up? A large order of fast-food fries ought to soothe those nerves. Feeling bored and antsy for no apparent reason at all? Assuage your jitters with some chips.

And why not? Food is legal, it's widely available, and it's—well, it's tasty. Goodies also hearken back to the comforting days when your mother would take you for an ice cream cone to lift your mood after a visit to the pediatrician for shots.

But it's a vicious circle: chowing down on goodies when you're bored, anxious or stressed can pile on the pounds, which in turn makes you feel even more stressed. There's another physical reason we find comfort in snacking when we're stressed: Cortisol is released by our bodies as part of the "fight or flight" response to stress. And cortisol stimulates the appetite, especially for carbohydrates.

But you don't have to let stress sabotage your healthy diet, instead:

- Reduce stress through lifestyle changes (reading this book is a good start!).
- Exercise regularly (see the Get a Move On! section, page 70, for more on exercise). Exercise encourages the release of endorphins—hormones

that fight stress, reduce cortisol levels and give you a sense of well-being.

- Give meditation a try. Like exercise, meditation encourages the release of endorphins.
- Have healthful, satisfying snacks ready to go so that you won't be tempted to reach for fatty fare when you're feeling stressed or anxious (or hungry!). Good choices include precut fruit, a handful of cashews or walnuts, or a slice of whole-grain bread with peanut butter and low-sugar preserves.
- Before you nosh, ask yourself if you're feeling stressed. If so, first take a quick walk, write in your journal or call a friend. Then decide whether you still want the snack.
- If you overindulge, think about why it happened, so you can plan ahead next time. Then let it go. Get back in touch with why it's important to take good care of yourself, and then get right back on track.
- Allow yourself small treats occasionally. Choosing a healthful diet you can live with in the long-term—including the occasional treat—will get you lifelong results. Fad or short-term diets can make you feel deprived, which can lead to bingeing—and they don't teach you to eat in a healthful manner for life.
- Cut back on sugar, caffeine and alcohol.

- Get your Zs. If you're not getting your eight hours every night, you'll feel anxious and run down. To enhance your slumber, make sure your bedroom is dark and cool. Go to bed at the same time every night, and get up at the same time every day—even on weekends.
- Get off to a good start! If you start your day with a Mountain Dew and a doughnut, you're on the fast track to stress eating. First of all, your blood sugar level will crash through the floor, causing stress and the temptation to gobble down those old Christmas candies that have been slowly melting in your desk drawer. Second, if you don't eat enough breakfast, your hunger will lead to overeating later in the day. So eat a small meal every three to four hours; this keeps your blood sugar level stable and your energy and focus up, all of which makes it much easier for you to deal with stress.

☼ *Think about . . .* my diet

When I'm stressed, I tend to crave:

1. _____

2. _____

3. _____

When I'm feeling stressed, instead of mindlessly snacking, I will:

__ Meditate

__ Exercise

__ Call a friend

__ Write in my journal

__ Use aromatherapy

__ Soak in the tub

__ Listen to some soothing tunes

Other: _____

_____

Think ahead to plan healthful snacks to replace less healthful things you might be tempted to snack on:

Instead of eating _____ (such as candy) when I'm feeling stressed, I'll snack on _____ (such as fruit).

Instead of eating _____ when I'm feeling stressed, I'll snack on _____.

Instead of eating _____ when I'm feeling stressed, I'll snack on _____.

Stress Tests

It felt like a velvet glove, moving up from my chest, spreading its fingers around my throat. The wild beating began then—this playing of a thousand notes up a xylophone. The tachycardia swelled like a symphony, until my heart was thudding like a runaway clock with stripped gears. I lay there and stared down at my thumping chest.

I'd just put my two young daughters to bed and had collapsed, exhausted, onto the bed I shared with my husband, who worked nights writing sports at the local newspaper. The strange episode passed, but the fright didn't. I waited up for him, talked into the wee hours. The next day we were sitting in the cardiologist's office and I went home wired up to a portable EKG machine I'd have to wear for three days.

"We've been over every beat," the doctor stated a week later. "There's no irregularity, but you do have a very significant mitral valve heart murmur. In time, it may need surgery, but for now, you just need to check in with me twice yearly. And for a young woman, you are in absolutely lousy shape!"

There began a reign of total terror now known as panic attacks. I got infected with the "fraids"—fraid of dying, fraid of leaving my children, fraid of having a heart attack. But what it really was, way down under, was massive stress. The stress of no money, mounting bills, no help from my husband who was always going out into his world of sports, dressed in a suit, traveling with the teams, while I stayed home twenty-four hours a day with tiny kids. And the big whammy—stress because I knew that my husband was systematically killing himself with three packs of cigarettes a day, fatty foods and a huge job that paid dividends in ego strokes, but was guaranteed to give him a stroke. I could be waiting at a traffic light, sitting alone evenings or in the middle of a crowd and the attacks swarmed over me like army ants. I didn't sleep much anymore because I was waiting to die. My digestion went south. Any food cranked off tremendous volcanic gastric explosions. Gasping for air, rolls of stomach gasses sent me into more panic because "what if" it really was a heart attack?

Most women weren't doing any exercise in the early seventies, and running was just making the scene. I bought a pair of two-dollar tennies, and one early morning, I took off running down the block in a skirt. Bent over and wheezing, I had to walk the second block. In a stop-start dog-and-pony show, ten blocks later, I got back to the house and met my perplexed husband and daughters waiting on the front porch.

"What *are* you doing?" LeRoy questioned, laughing.

"Running," I huffed, hobbling up the steps. "One more laugh, Bucko, and I'll smack you!"

Getting out of bed the next morning, I howled, then crumpled to the floor. My calves were molten fire. I had to lean on walls to get around. Two days later, I hobbled out there again. And so it went, again and again. In two months, I did my first real mile, nonstop. LeRoy wasn't laughing anymore. As the running grew stronger, panic and stress diminished. In 1974 I showed up for my first race in downtown Albuquerque, New Mexico, dressed in jeans, carrying a purse. When the starting horn blared, I shoved it into my cardiologist's hands. Forty-eight minutes later, LeRoy, the girls and the doc, who was swinging my purse like artillery, cheered me in—first four miles ever, twelve-minute pace, back of the pack. I was hooked.

Two years later I became a widow. LeRoy died at forty-two of a totally wrecked heart. His arteries were in shreds from genetics, from smoking, from fats and from stress. Time passed. Wounded hearts healed—my daughters' and mine. I remarried.

For twenty-eight years I ran half-marathons over roads, hills, mountains and American byways. I made every part of this beautiful big-hearted country mine on foot. Sunrise found me on the Grand Canyon rim, Missouri paths, Houston bayous and the Mississippi River at New Orleans where I heard the mournful song of a sunrise sax. My heart swelled for the beauty of it all—this country passing under my thudding feet, trampling stress, breathing in wisdom and life. I was like a train, speeding through hot flashes, cheapo eyeglasses, graying hair, winning medals, doing seven-minute miles. The kids grew up, the dogs died. I got checked, my EKGs read, but no doc ever said I was in lousy shape again.

When I got bumped to another health care program, three strange docs watched the computer screen as I ran the treadmill.

"Are you on beta blockers?" one asked cautiously, while reviewing my super-low blood pressure and the odd, slow spike with a kick heart blip that comes with athletics.

"Nah," I replied casually. "Been running twenty-eight years, and I quit dressing other people."

"Hardly any blood is leaking back in the mitral valve," reported doc number two.

"Dressing others?" queried the third.

"I quit trying to dress other people in my dreams,

fears and desires," I said wistfully, continuing my slow jog. "What is, is. I do what I can, and I let go of the rest."

"No problema with this thumper," said number two with a huge smile. "Get the heck outta here, lady jock! You got the secret of life!"

Long ago, I came to accept that if I died, I died. But to live in fear, or to live not giving my absolute personal best every day was a life not worth living. These days, at nearly seventy, I walk with my husband, do aerobics faithfully with all of the young flat-bellies in my class, and occasionally run a mile for old time's sake in the cool of an Albuquerque foothills sunrise, when I see my mountain rising out of lavender mist and a good city yawning itself awake.

♥ *Isabel Bearman Bucher*

Get a Move On!
Beating Stress Through Exercise

Exercise is one of the best ways to combat stress and stress eating. Exercise increases endorphins in your body, which trigger happiness, tranquility and a sense of well-being. And it's as easy as taking a walk!

If the word *exercise* conjures up an image of leotard-clad women sweating to the exhortations of a bubbly, aerobicized fitness instructor, don't worry. Exercise also includes such fun activities as karate, Pilates and swimming. But the best exercise to do is the type you'll do every day or almost every day. Walking for half an hour a day is better than working out in the gym for two hours once a week, for example. So pick something you can do regularly, and stick with it.

Follow these tips to get your body moving, get your blood pumping and blast your stress:

- Choose something you can commit to on a daily or every-other-day basis.
- Keep it simple. Walking, doing yoga with a video at home or riding a bicycle to work are great ways to take care of yourself.
- Have an exercise buddy to make sure you stick with the program—even a dog will do!

- Make a six-week commitment to your choice of exercise to see if it's a good fit for you. It takes about that long to create a habit, and once your exercise routine is a habit, you don't have to decide every day whether or not to do it—it will be automatic.
- If you miss a day, don't dwell on it. Just get back into the habit the following day. Don't let one missed day become a missed week.
- Skip the workout if you're feeling rundown or getting sick. Your body needs all its energy to cope with the threat to your health.
- Break up your exercise into shorter blocks if you need to on some days. Walk up the stairs at work during a break, park far from your destination when you run an errand, or vacuum your house. Once you get in the habit of adding these quick exercise fixes, you may find you can add them to your daily routine.

CHOOSING A GYM

If you're the type of person who finds it motivating to exercise in a group, you'll want to look into joining a gym, the local Y or a hospital-affiliated wellness program. You don't have to spend a lot of money to find a nice, clean place to exercise—many communities have low-cost community centers offering a gym and workout classes. Don't choose a facility that's too far away—you may be motivated to go now, but will you still want to drive there three times a week next winter? Is the facility's schedule convenient for you? Visit at the time of day you're most likely to go when you're a member. See whether there's a long wait for the equipment you want to use. Make sure there are classes geared to your ability level. Are there staff members available to show you how to correctly use the equipment?

GET A NUTRITIOUS START

Just as your car needs fuel to drive, your body needs fuel to exercise. Here are some tips to get you started:

- Always eat a breakfast that includes filling whole grains, cereals and fruits. This is important even on the days you are not exercising.
- Ideally, several hours before you work out, eat a balanced meal containing carbohydrates, fats and protein—such as whole-grain bread with sliced turkey, condiments and 2 percent milk, or an all-natural peanut butter sandwich on whole-grain bread accompanied by a salad topped with olive oil vinaigrette or yogurt, or a whole-wheat pasta dish topped with tomato sauce and lean ground meat.
- If you aren't able to plan that far ahead, snack

on foods half an hour or so ahead of time that are lower in fat and easily digested so that you have enough energy for your workout—good choices would be fruit; high-fiber, all-natural crackers; low-fat cottage cheese; skim milk or a small turkey breast sandwich on whole-grain bread.

- Always drink plenty of water before, during and after your workout to prevent your muscles from becoming cramped or sore.

Ask Your Doctor

Be sure to consult with your doctor before starting an exercise program if any of the following apply:

- You are a man over 40 or a woman over 50.
- You have a heart condition.
- You feel discomfort in your chest when you do physical activity.
- You ever become dizzy or lose your balance.
- You have a bone or joint problem.
- You are diabetic.
- You take blood pressure or heart medications.

Think about . . .
moving my body

What do I need to do before I get started on an exercise program?

__ See my doctor

__ Buy quality sneakers and workout clothes

__ Find a workout partner

__ Buy a workout video

__ Buy exercise equipment

Other: _____

_____

_____

I'll start with this type of exercise every day or every other day:

__ Weight training and cardio at the gym

__ Yoga

__ Martial arts

__ Walking

__ Dance

__ Swimming

__ Biking

Other: _____

_____

_____

When I get bored with my exercise routine, I will:

__ Keep showing up so I don't disappoint my exercise buddy.

__ Use music to get in the mood.

__ Plan a treat for when I reach a goal (for example, I'll treat myself to a massage if I exercise regularly for two months).

__ Vary my workouts by mixing in other types of exercise.

Other: _____

_____

_____

My notes:

_____

_____

Type A Mind, Type B Body

I had failed. I had never left a job in my entire career due to illness, until now.

It started with not being able to sleep at night, and when I did, it was a fitful, restless slumber. I was having indigestion and raging bouts of diarrhea. I couldn't concentrate, hardly went a week without a crushing migraine and spent lots of hours at the chiropractor getting "unkinked." I had lost twenty pounds in a year that I didn't need to lose.

Then one day I just couldn't go on; my energy was zapped, and I was a mess. Tears rolled down my cheeks as I dotted the "i" in Sallie as I signed my resignation letter. How did it come to this?

At first, I didn't understand what was happening to me. I thought I was just going through a bad phase. For two years, I had put twelve hours worth of work into eight hour days, and my body had finally cried out for mercy.

One night not long after leaving my job, my eldest daughter called.

"Mom, are you in bed with a headache again?" she asked.

"Yeah, I just can't seem to shake these migraines. It's like my body is giving out, but my mind still wants to go, go, go."

"Maybe you're a type A personality in a type B body," she declared.

I started to laugh. *What a funny way to put it,* I thought.

That night I lay awake in bed as the clock ticked away the hours. I began thinking about what my daughter had said. *She may have a point,* I conceded. I was barely fifty and had worked my entire life for high-powered CEOs and presidents of companies, thriving on the fast-paced atmosphere. I had always enjoyed the pace, but it wasn't fun anymore. I wanted more balance in my life, time to smell the roses. My body was sending me an SOS, and I needed to listen.

The next day I made another doctor's appointment. He had seen a lot of me lately and the diagnosis was always the same—stress. Now I wanted to know how I could climb out of this hole I had created. I told him I had quit my stressful job but would need to go back to work eventually. I asked him what he thought I should do. He suggested some blood tests, a colonoscopy and some cancer tests to rule out serious problems.

I ran through the tests with flying colors but dragged through the days with no energy. After several visits, Western medicine had pretty much given all it could give.

The doctor told me, "Your period of prolonged stress has caused irritable bowel syndrome (IBS). It's chronic; you'll just have to learn to live with it. Your quality of life may suffer some. Try different approaches. You'll know what works after some trial and error. That's about all you can do."

Stunned, mad and determined not to give up, I turned to Eastern medicine. I found a holistic practitioner who prescribed nutrients, vitamins and minerals. For a year, I took easy-to-digest supplements, digestive enzymes, napped a lot, read and generally relaxed. Then came the day I knew was inevitable. I needed to return to work.

I found a low-key job and slowly worked my way back into the routine. I left the job at work when I went home at five o'clock. I didn't look back or lie awake all night. I gradually gained some energy and managed my IBS as well as I could. Some days were tougher than others, but I never missed a day of work from it.

It has been four years since I signed that resignation letter. I am working again for a government official, but I have learned to deal with stress and pace myself. I take vitamins and Chinese herbs, consult with my regular doctor once a year and meditate regularly. I can't do aerobics, yet, as I'm still trying to gain back all my weight, but I have taken up t'ai chi to still my type A mind. Someday soon I'll be at the gym; until then, I walk for exercise. Oh, I still get an occasional bout of IBS. That's when I ask myself what's stressing me, and I deal with it immediately. Prolonged stress manifests in many ways; mine happens to be IBS.

Am I sorry that all this happened to me? Not at all. I am much happier and well-rounded. The experience taught me the value of listening to my body, loving my body, balancing my life and addressing stress before it causes an illness. My type B body is happier, too.

♥ *Sallie A. Rodman*

Cop an Attitude!

Have you ever said that someone has an attitude problem? Well, you may be more right than you think: A person's attitude toward life and living can cause stress and anxiety. A small adjustment to your attitude can mean the difference between feeling stressed all the time and living life to its fullest. Don't think a bad attitude can happen to you? Here are some questions to contemplate when you have at least ten to fifteen minutes of uninterrupted time. (Tip: Turn off the TV, and don't answer the phone.)

1. How much of your stress is caused by your approach to life? Review the quiz on page 6 and find out how your stress style keeps you feeling stressed.

2. How much of your stress is caused by bad habits that you've fallen into? Are you spending too much money so that you have to work more overtime? Do you say things you regret later? Does your drinking or drug use lead to regrettable or embarrassing behavior?

3. How much of your stress is caused by the way you react to problems that come up in your day-to-day life? Do you get too little sleep so that you overreact to minor stressors? Do you put yourself in bad situations you could have

avoided because you naively hope things will turn out differently?

Try these tips to help you change your attitude and blast your stress:

- Live by your most cherished values. It's very stressful to act differently from what you believe is right.
- Don't let yourself feel like a victim. The more helpless you feel, the more stress you allow into your life.
- Don't overestimate what you can control. Accept what you can't control, and don't waste energy worrying about things that have nothing to do with you. (See page 52 for more on this.)
- Develop an *attitude of gratitude*. Give thanks every day for all that's going well in your life. Write down your thoughts and feelings, and review your "Gratitude Journal" when you're feeling down. You can even teach your children to make this a habit by asking them to recount one thing each day—at dinner or before they go to sleep are good times—that they are grateful for.
- Use music to change your mood for the better. We're wired as humans to respond to music. That's why movies use soundtracks—they set a

tone and create a mood. What do you find uplifting? Put it on!

- Do the most important task in the beginning of your day whenever possible. That way, if you get interrupted or run out of time or energy mid-day, you won't have to stress about not doing something that really needed to get done.

Think about . . .
my attitude

Here are some ways I can give myself an "attitude adjustment":

__ Put on inspiring music, such as _____.

__ Pick one essential task each day and get it done early. Today I'll: _____.

__ Learn to accept what I can't change. This will require some contemplation on my part!

__ Start a "Gratitude Journal." I'll start now by listing three things I'm grateful for today:

_____

_____

_____

__ Live according to what I believe is right. This might mean putting my children ahead of my social obligations, volunteering for a cause I believe in or not passing along juicy gossip.

__ Stop feeling like a victim, stop taking things too personally, and try to find the humor in life's minor challenges.

All in the Family

Nobody wanted to be there. Not even one person. However, they were all there, and in a strange way, glad they were. This was the waiting room of the Neuro Trauma Intensive Care Unit (NTICU) at Memorial Hermann Hospital, one of only two "level one trauma hospitals" in Houston, Texas.

The first few days, as a rule, the families keep to themselves. However, as time passes by, the families usually get to know each other—they share the joy when there is good news for a family, and they also share the sorrow when there is poor news for a family.

The unit's many families become a "support group" for each other. I have seen it often. As one of the social workers for the hospital, I understand the dynamics of hope and the importance of support. I have seen families volunteer to take a family from out-of-town to their homes so that they could rest and shower. I have also seen strangers pray for the recovery of someone whom they did not even know twenty-four hours earlier.

There are many miraculous stories about the

families in the NTICU. Unfortunately, there are
many times when there is not a happy ending. On
one occasion, a young man was severely hurt and
suffered a traumatic brain injury, and he was
rushed to our hospital. For days, his prognosis was
in doubt. His mother was always in the waiting
room, and I am sure she experienced a roller coaster
of emotions. Of course, she breathed a huge sigh of
relief when the doctors gave her reason to hope.

Then she saw another mother in the waiting
room whose daughter had not been given that
hopeful prognosis. The daughter, she was told by
the doctors, would probably soon pass away as a
result of the severe injuries that she had sustained
in a car accident.

The two mothers were soon linked together—
strangers joined forever by a universal magnet,
mothers' pain. They became very close, supporting
each other in both good and bad times.

Ironically, the predictions for the two mothers
were eventually reversed. The young man, who was
supposed to survive, unfortunately passed away,
while the girl who was supposed to die is now making progress at home in California.

In another case, there were two patients—an elderly gentleman and a teenager—who had been in
the NTICU for quite some time. Their families got
to know each other and became close.

The parents of the teenager were at the hospital night and day. But one night, the teenager's mother returned to her home while his father remained in the waiting room. The next morning she returned to the hospital and said to the wife of the elderly patient, who regularly remained at the hospital night and day also, "I was worried about you all night."

The elderly woman responded, "I figured you were worried, because last night I was sleeping with your husband in the waiting room, and I wouldn't have missed it for the world!"

Everyone burst out in deep laughter. Humor can be a great coping mechanism.

♥ *Michael Jordan Segal, MSW*

Don't Fly Solo: Support Systems

Does coping with stress seem like a personal, solitary effort? After all, busting stress means changing your dietary habits, which can alienate friends who are used to having you as an ice cream parlor or happy hour partner. And taking time to exercise and practice self-care means you have less time to take on special projects at work, which may not make your boss and co-workers too happy.

It feels like a lonely job, but in reality you need the support of others to beat stress. Explain to the people you know and love that you're making an effort to reduce your stress and get healthy, and that you need their support. Be sure to point out that a less-stressed you will be a lot more fun to be with!

People who have more personal connections tend to suffer less from depression and stress. We all need someone to talk to when we're feeling overwhelmed! But many of us find that our hectic lives don't allow us to develop close, interdependent relationships. Now is the time to change these habits. Join a club, start a new hobby or volunteer for a cause you believe in—you're sure to meet people who share your mind-set.

STRESS AND PETS

Even Fido or Fluffy can help you de-stress! Many people find that interacting with a pet makes them feel more relaxed and content. Some researchers claim benefits such as reduced blood pressure. Do you have a pet? If so, what activities might you find relaxing to do with it?

__ Brushing or petting your dog or cat
__ Reading a book with your cat or your dog at your feet (or on your chest)
__ Sleeping with your pet
__ Going to obedience class with your dog to help be part of your family's life and less stressful to live with
__ Taking regular walks with your dog
__ Taking your dog to the dog park (This is also a great way to meet people!)
__ Throwing a ball or playing with pet toys together
__ Bringing your pet to visit an ill or disabled neighbor or friend (or getting involved with a pet-assisted therapy group)

Keep in mind that while many people find having a pet relaxing and can't imagine life without one, others find it stressful to be responsible for a pet. And if you're too busy to care properly for a pet, it isn't fair to the animal. (And we don't need to tell you that getting a pet for a child means that the parent will be the real caretaker!)

☀ Think about . . .
my support system

Here's where I can get the support I need to make lasting lifestyle changes:

__ Friends and family members

__ Church, temple or other spiritual center

__ Classes related to a hobby or interest

__ Professional association, trade association

__ Parenting or school-related organization (moms' club, PTA or Tough Love) or an after-school association (like Scouts)

__ A neighbor you'd like to know better

__ A reputable volunteer organization you believe in

__ Online groups or lists related to an interest, hobby or medical condition

__ A dog or cat

December Dreamer

Always a dreamer, I longed for a white Christmas, just like the ones in Chicago, my Midwest birth city. The past two Christmases my midwestern snowy dreams came true, but sandwiched between was a pile of stressors.

My stress was triggered at 8:15 A.M., Friday the thirteenth of February, in southwest Pennsylvania. My husband often called during the workday to encourage a break in my writing. Usually Andy's voice was a daily hug, but that Friday voice frightened me as I asked him to repeat what he had said.

"I was just laid off from the company," he said, adding, "Seventeen and a half years, and I can never enter the gates again."

Life cascaded into numbered agonies and ecstasies—or distresses, bad stressors, and "eustresses," good stressors, as coined by Dr. Hans Selye, the father of stress research.

Three of them were our kids. Michael, our eldest, worried he wasted our money attending out-of-state Ohio State University. Daughter Jessica jotted scriptures and cheerful quotes for Dad; still, she was distracted in her community college courses. And our youngest was sixteen going on five; Peter was high functioning, yet cognitively challenged from past seizures.

Meanwhile, 454 miles west the kids' grandmother, Andy's delightful mom, Dee, was not responding to chemotherapy.

How it hurt as I urged Andy out of bed that first unemployed week. I was a bucket weeper; Andy was a guy. I watched his thick fingers press into his tear ducts to stop two tears. The next nine weeks Andy job searched, exercised, job searched. He lost twenty pounds. We all lost countless hours of sleep. We curtailed expenses by eating at home and shopping less.

On Good Friday a company in Dayton, Ohio, presented Andy a job offer. Dayton was nearer to OSU and nearer to Andy's parents! We visited Dayton, touring fifty homes in two days, settling on a house with only a foundation on a street under construction.

I captained the cleaning, moving and selling of the old house while Andy lived fifty days at a hotel near his new job and ten weekends at home. We both gained the weight he lost—and more.

In the muddle of stressors Andy's mom had renal failure. So we rushed to hug her. The day before

Mother's Day, Dee sailed painlessly into eternal rest.

We moved in July. Adrenaline pumped, I emp-
tied forty-five boxes the day we moved, and the next
three months made the house beautiful through the
din of neighborhood construction. The final distress: After six seizure-free years, dear Peter had a
seizure on the school bus in November.

Christmas Day snowfall quilted beauty over the
surrounding construction mess. But snow couldn't
hide the mess of me. Mornings I woke to migraines.
Nights my arms tingled. My heart burned pain. My
eyes burned salty. Clothes felt tight. I couldn't write
much. Through the holidays, my honey urged me
to see a doctor.

January second I met trim Dr. Manahan, who
said, "Please, call me Jill." In a New York minute I
rattled off the chronology of stressors to Dr. Jill.
Together we formulated a treatment strategy. First I
went for a blood test to see if thyroid imbalances
held me hostage to calories and mood bends.
Thankfully, the results were negative. Medication
was the next consideration. As a writer I needed my
senses clear, not dulled.

Dr. Jill thought a year on a low dose of Zoloft
would be helpful for me; she said the fog of adjustment would be short-lived. Also, I restarted my
daily purple pill to combat stress-triggered acid
reflux.

Next we discussed holistic treatments. Jill asked
if I had found a good church. I told her I had—
Emmanuel Lutheran, Kettering. Church had helped
our family survive 2004. Church support would
help us again. I also needed exercise motivation. Dr.
Jill gave me the green light to join the local YMCA,
so the family joined. Fitness counselor Kevin eased
me into a regular cardio-fitness/weight-loss regime.
Jill added, "If you need to—call me." It was thera-
peutic having my doctor be a friend.

After a week and a half of fog, I was able to fill
my iBook screen with one-thousand-word stories;
my former output was four hundred. Exercise, I
learned, was fun when you're moving with others.
Cardio-aerobics seemed to sweat away stress adrenaline. The tingles, heart pains and frenzied hyper-
anxiety diminished.

As for tears, they fall, but I don't need buckets to
collect them. Now that life for my family is stressor-
less, we're dreaming of an upbeat Christmas—with
or without the white stuff.

♥ *Cynthia Hinkle*

Turning to a Pro

If the "check engine" light went on in your car, you'd probably take the car in to a pro. But most of us, when we're feeling stressed, ignore our own "check engine" lights—like headaches, irritability or other symptoms of stress.

Many of us are reluctant to "bother" our doctor when we have emotional or physical symptoms that we believe are due to stress. But even for the strong, silent types, it's important to let our physician know about changes in our health, no matter what the cause or trigger.

Consult with your physician and mention the stressors in your life.

Pointing out that you're stressed isn't a way of minimizing your physical symptoms. Physical symptoms triggered by stress are not "all in your head."

WHO SHOULD I SEE?

Your doctor may suggest that you consult with a psychiatrist, psychologist or psychotherapist. But what's the difference—and which will be most helpful to you?

A **psychiatrist** (MD) is a physician who has been to medical school, has special training, and is licensed by the state in diagnosing and treating psychiatric conditions. A psychiatrist is the only mental health professional who can prescribe psychiatric medication if needed. (Your internist or any other medical doctor can also prescribe psychiatric medication.)

Many psychiatrists only diagnose psychiatric disorders, treat them with medication and monitor the effects of the medication. Others provide psychotherapy.

A **psychologist** (PhD or PsyD) has a doctorate degree in psychology, as well as a state psychology license. They have special training in diagnosing psychiatric conditions, and most offer psychotherapy services. Some psychologists specialize in certain areas, while others treat a wide variety of clients.

A **mental health counselor** (MA or MSW) has a master's degree and a state license to practice counseling. They have training in psychotherapy techniques, including diagnosing and treating a variety of conditions. Many have specialty areas related to working with families and children.

CHOOSING A PROFESSIONAL

A psychiatrist is able to diagnose and treat a patient with these symptoms:

• Depression, including sadness, a feeling of

"deadness," sleep disorders, weight loss or gain
- Hearing voices
- Altered states of consciousness (not related to drug or alcohol use)
- Abuse of drugs or alcohol
- Manic states (needing less sleep, increased amount of energy, poor judgment including spending large amounts of money, being sexually promiscuous, or other risky behaviors)
- Suicidal thoughts or attempts

A psychologist or a mental health counselor can treat someone with the above symptoms (in some cases only if they are on medication prescribed by a psychiatrist or other physician). They can also treat the following, depending on their areas of expertise:

- Stress (including post-traumatic stress disorder)
- Family conflicts, including separation, divorce, and parent-child relationship problems
- Disorders such as ADD or ADHD
- Grief
- Coping with the emotional aspects of a disability or chronic illness

Psychologists can provide psychological testing, which can be a useful tool for diagnosing psychiatric conditions. Counselors are more likely to be skilled at treating families, children and adolescents.

Typically, psychiatrists charge the most per hour, and psychologists usually charge more than counselors. Whichever type of professional you choose, interview him or her to make sure you feel comfortable before beginning treatment.

PROFESSIONAL SUPPORT GROUPS

Previously we discussed how important it is to get support from your extended family, your community and other people or nonprofessional groups. Now we'll talk about groups run by a trained professional.

Professional support groups are especially useful when you're in need of support for a condition with serious symptoms or when a facilitator would be helpful to keep the group focused, resolve conflicts, provide information or encourage introspection.

Issues that professionally run support groups can help you with include:

- Loss and grief
- Divorce
- Preparation for marriage
- Chronic illness
- Infertility
- Parenting
- Men's, women's, or teens' issues

Many professionally run groups can be found listed in your local newspaper. Or check local hospitals, community centers, churches and temples. You can also do an Internet search for a specific topic if you're having trouble finding a group in your area. (There are also online groups or lists that can be very helpful, although these are rarely run by a professional.)

Note: Be wary of irresponsible professionals and others in your growing support system who are content to complain and to stay stuck where they are. Keep searching until you find the right match for you.

Professionals should have wisdom to go along with their credentials.

Groups should offer hope as well as information. And as they say at the end of many 12-step meetings, "It works if you work it!"

MEDICATIONS

Although your internist can prescribe psychiatric medications, it often makes sense to consult a psychiatrist because they diagnose and treat psychiatric conditions with medication full-time.

When medication is indicated, many conditions (like depression) respond best to a combination of medication and individual or group psychotherapy. You can go to a psychiatrist for medication and a psychologist or counselor for psychotherapy. Or you can go to a psychiatrist who does both medication monitoring and psychotherapy.

Many medication options exist, and your doctor may try a particular medication for a period of time to see if you benefit from it. If you don't, or if you have unpleasant side effects, he or she may try a different medication. Follow instructions and keep track of all side effects to help your doctor make the best recommendations for you.

Take all medication exactly as prescribed. Let your doctor know about side effects between visits if necessary, rather than altering the dose on your own.

Ask your doctor about drinking alcoholic beverages, or other dietary restrictions, while on a particular medication. And ask if you have other restrictions, such as driving, while starting a new medication.

☼ *Think about . . .*
whether I should see a professional

I'm experiencing these symptoms:

__ Chest pains

__ Trouble sleeping

__ Changes in my appetite or weight

__ Anxiety, irritability, sadness, a "dead" feeling or lack of enjoyment of things I usually enjoy

__ Exhaustion, frequent illness, feeling run-down much of the time

__ Stomach upset, cramping, diarrhea or constipation

__ Headaches, migraines, jaw pain, back or neck aches or spasms

__ Worsening of an ongoing condition, including skin conditions

Meditation—The Best Medication

Juggling appointments, scheduling consultations, babysitting, setting aside time for writing, and all the daily chores that keep a household running smoothly can be so overwhelming. To help me cope, I would meditate every Friday with friends. It was the one day I felt calm and could wade through the storm of my stressful week. One Friday during meditation, a voice came from within. It told me that I would go through much suffering, but would not die. I told my friends what my meditation revealed, but eventually dismissed it as not being real.

Soon after, I found myself on an operating schedule for open-heart surgery to replace a faulty heart valve. While I waited for my date with the knife, I went for a second opinion. That physician diagnosed cardiomyopathy, an enlargement of the heart muscle, and confidently informed me that I did not need the operation, after all.

I had mixed emotions. I was relieved, yet still concerned. I also had this nagging pain in my abdomen. My new cardiologist sent me for a CAT scan, which is when the bombshell hit. In spite of routine biannual checkups, one very recently when I was assured that everything was fine, I had ovarian cancer. I was in disbelief. I was more than angry; I was enraged!

After having a complete hysterectomy, I went through the stages of grief. My heart was stronger than the doctors thought, but I needed something more to get me through. My family and friends were very supportive; still it wasn't enough. My stress barometer was past anxiety—it was inching up to pure fear. I knew I was going to die.

"Calm down," a voice inside whispered, "You will not die. . . ." Then I heard, "Meditate." I took some cleansing breaths and began to sit quietly.

For the first time, I realized that heart failure and cardiomyopathy had saved my life. If my cardiologist hadn't sent me for that CAT scan, the ovarian cancer would have gone undetected. I guess I always knew, deep down, on a subconscious level, that I would recover. I made a vow—never doubt my meditations again.

I have replaced worry with awe. I no longer juggle a daily schedule; whatever I choose to do gets done joyfully. I don't live for Friday anymore; I live for now. A double dose of awakening was much more profound than all the medicine and chemotherapy that keeps my heart functioning and the cancer at bay.

But there's something more. It's called Faith, with a capital "F." Living with cardiomyopathy and cancer is an intimate challenge. They eat, sleep and breathe with me. Even when everything is going well, they remind me how precious life is. Because I now believe that my health is a gift, I am not consumed with fear. I will not let cancer take over my identity, and most important, I will not think about "what's going to happen next." I know I'm not a defective heart or a cell gone awry. Both may live in me, but they're not the core of who I am.

Now I *meditate* daily; it's how I begin to *medicate.* There's only one letter difference between the two words, yet *meditation* is my best *medication*; it's my prescription for happiness.

♥ *Dolores Kozielski*

Stress and Spirituality

Sometimes, when we're feeling stressed, it's hard to get outside of our own heads, which buzz with negative thoughts and worries. That's why an important aspect to reducing stress is to contemplate something higher than ourselves. Knowing that our lives have a purpose (even if we don't fully understand what it is yet) and understanding that we're a small part of a vast universe can take a lot of pressure off us.

THE POWER OF PRAYER

For some, the way to get in touch with something higher than ourselves is through a religious or traditional spiritual practice. For others, it is through a personal connection with God or a higher power.

Having a religious or spiritual practice that you incorporate into your daily life may be one of the most powerful ways to reduce stress and find life more meaningful and satisfying.

Do you pray? If so, how might you use the power of prayer to help you cope with stress?

MEDITATION

Another way to tune in to your true self and to de-stress is to meditate, or as some would say, to enter into your inner silence. This involves being fully present in the moment and in touch with your soul—the divine spark in all of us. There are many ways to do this: You can take a class, listen to a CD or read a book about meditating.

Meditating even ten minutes a day, preferably at the same time each day, can have profound benefits, such as:

- Lowered blood pressure
- The ability to observe your reactions to stressful events more objectively and with detachment
- A feeling of peace and calm

It takes practice, so don't be discouraged if you don't feel calm and peaceful right away. In fact, you'll probably feel a bit bored or distracted until you break through the initial resistance to quieting your active mind. Follow these tips to get off to a good start:

- Set aside a special place in your home to pray or meditate.
- Be consistent.
- Set realistic goals for how long you'll meditate.
- Turn off the TV, phone, radio and computer, and try to get used to having more quiet, reflective time.
- Teach your children to meditate, or do yoga with them.

- Practice observing your reaction to others, to stressors and even to positive things like compliments. Try to stretch out the moment of time between a stimulus and your reaction to it. In other words, think before you react!

Healer: Yoga

The physical practice of yoga was developed thousands of years ago by practitioners of the spiritual practice of yoga (meaning those "yoking" themselves to God) as a way to prepare their bodies and minds for meditation. There are many who see yoga as a way to get in great shape or stay flexible, and it does work well as an exercise. But the physical exercise of yoga (or "hatha yoga") is still a wonderful way to focus and calm your mind, quiet your thoughts and prepare your body to sit in meditation.

Think about . . .
my spiritual practice

Here's what I'll do to focus more on my spirit—
and become less stressed:

__ Meditate ten to twenty minutes each day.

__ Take a meditative walk. Some people chant a
mantra or focus on their breathing while
walking. This is called "walking meditation."

__ Pray according to my religious beliefs.

__ Post a picture or a quote in a prominent place
to remind me to turn toward God or my
higher power when I get caught up in my hectic daily activities.

__ Read from a spiritual text or other inspirational material in the morning or at bedtime.

__ Listen to a tape or CD on a spiritual or uplifting topic.

__ Do yoga before meditating to quiet my body
and mind.

Don't Smell the Roses

I cannot remember what exactly got me to a point of complete exhaustion and feeling overwhelmed with my day-to-day routine, but I do know that I definitely reached that point. I tried using a grocery delivery service, simplifying dinners and having a housekeeper clean my house once a week, but still I was left feeling too busy to take time to enjoy life and truly feel happy.

Something had to give, but at this point, I was unaware that it might just be me. Desperate to find a way to enjoy life without selling my house and moving my family to a remote log cabin far away from a modern lifestyle, I decided to entertain the New-Age adage, "we create our own reality." I also embraced a new mantra, "it does not have to be perfect."

I put this recipe for change to the test. I decided that there would be enough time to take one hour, three days per week to put everything on hold and use my exercise equipment before making dinner. The results were astonishing; nobody starved or even suffered from eating dinner at seven rather than at six. Furthermore, I found that I actually smiled while I prepared dinner for my family after working out.

Finding the time to do housework has always been difficult for me. My house is always clean and perhaps at times close to sterile. My newly created reality is now to settle for clean enough. Everything that gets cleaned in three hours is all that gets cleaned; everything else can wait until the next week. Since this new routine has been in effect, I am pleased to report the house looks just as good as it did when I would spend an entire day making sure I did not miss a spot.

The list of examples of how I have created a new reality in everyday life could go on and on. However, I have decided that this story does not have to be perfect, and I do not have to spend much time to get my thoughts across. In summary, only a few short months ago, I did not have the time to exercise, walk my child to school rather than having him take the bus, keep up with the laundry or go grocery shopping.

Since adopting the philosophy of creating my own reality (yes, the glass remains half full) and remembering that it doesn't have to be perfect, I exercise, walk my child to school and no longer need a housekeeper or a grocery delivery service. I have more time, or at least I choose to see things that way.

Will I take time to smell the roses? Only if they are in somebody else's yard. Planting roses this year is something I don't really need to do to feel happy. I'll settle for taking time to smell the pansies that somehow popped up all over my yard this year.

♥ *Shirley Warren*

*"Our life is frittered away by detail. . . .
Simplify, simplify, simplify!"*

—HENRY DAVID THOREAU

Keep It Simple, Sweetie!
Simplify Your Life Without
Feeling Deprived

Your living room looks like an explosion at JCPenney. You can't find the recipe that you clipped last week, not to mention your phone bill, the stamps or your car keys. No wonder you're stressed out!

Clutter adds to our stress. Similarly, an organized and attractive home or office with open space makes us feel more relaxed and comfortable, with fewer worries that something important will slip through the cracks—or get buried in a pile.

To paraphrase the comedian George Carlin, our stuff is "stuff" but someone else's stuff is "junk." It's hard to get rid of our "stuff," and it's even harder to stop bringing more of it home.

Let's break this down into three parts:

1. Value having less stuff.

Make sure your spouse or partner and children are on the same page with you. Focus on the positives: Your spouse may appreciate that you'll save money, and the house will be less cluttered. Young children want what they want, but they'll also emulate you to some extent. Older children and teens can begin to appreciate the value in living a simpler life.

It's especially important to focus on the positive aspects of simplifying your life with your children, as opposed to focusing on what you, or they, can't have. If you have less debt, you won't have to work as much overtime and can spend more time with them. You can start a habit of having a weekly game night at home instead of going out to dinner and a movie each week. In these ways, simplifying your life can enhance your quality of life in ways your children can appreciate.

2. Get rid of existing stuff.

If you live with others, don't be too quick to get rid of their "junk." Set an example by sorting through your "stuff" first. Again, make this a positive experience for your family by making a game of seeing who can find the most items to get rid of and donating items in good condition to charity. Ask your children to choose a few toys or stuffed animals they no longer play with, and bring them with you to a children's hospital or charity where they can see the grateful recipients, if possible.

The hardest part of getting rid of our stuff is that we get emotionally attached to these things. How can I get rid of the ill-fitting and unflattering shirt my late, beloved grandfather gave me? Other times, there is a social obligation involved. What if my mother-in-law looks for the tea set she gave me two Christmases ago? Follow these tips on letting go of your stuff:

- Instead of coming up with a reason to donate or toss something, make yourself come up with a reason to keep it.
- Have a box or pile for things you're not sure what to do with. This way, you don't default to keeping something that you're not sure about.
- When you go into a room, find one thing to throw away or donate. Go through a file, pick a book from the shelf, or go through the kitchen utility drawer.

3. Stop bringing in more stuff.

Once you've gotten rid of a significant amount of stuff, it's time to protect your newly organized home or office. If you delay an impulse purchase, there's a good chance you won't buy that item. And if you do buy it, it will probably be a smarter decision. So before you buy something, try these tips to engage your brain before you open your wallet:

- Keep a list of things you'd like to buy and review it every month. You'll probably cross most things off the list before buying them.
- If you do need an item, take the time to do some research so you get the best value. You'll be less likely to have buyer's remorse, and you'll discover the "cons" before you're stuck with the item.
- Don't believe the hype. Will that tiny vacuum

cleaner that looks so handy actually pick up pet hair like in the commercial? Or will you still use your full-size vacuum cleaner and toss the smaller one in the back of the closet?

- Ask yourself: Can I live without it? Do I already own something similar?
- If your weakness is shopping for your child, always needing a new pocketbook, or having to upgrade your stereo equipment, keep a list of what you need and a separate list of what you want. Use the latter for special occasions only.

☼ Think about . . .
simplifying my life

What ten things can I cut out of my life?

1. _____

2. _____

3. _____

4. _____

5. _____

6. _____

7. _____

8. _____

9. _____

10. _____

From Stress to Serenity

The summer of 1986. With so many things in my life going right, fate played a cruel joke. I had been setting up educational material for therapists on the devastation of child abuse, counseling families impacted by cancer and working with adults experiencing anxiety disorders. I loved the excitement of learning new things, as well as reaching out into the community to be of service.

Then it happened. I started to get very tired. At first I thought it was a bug of some kind. I began to take extra vitamin C, garlic and echinacea along with my regular vitamins. I visualized healing light around my body. I pushed myself to exercise as much as I could. I prayed hard. After two months, I gave up and dragged myself to the doctor.

"You have a bad case of chronic fatigue syndrome," Dr. Brown said after the blood tests came back. "It can develop from a multiplicity of factors that we don't have control of. Stress lowers the immune system and makes us all susceptible to illness."

"Stress?"

He nodded and looked away. "There isn't anything I can do. Just rest and do what you can. Chronic fatigue can take five years to get out of your system."

I was stunned. What had I done to deserve this terrible illness?

At the end of the first year, I could barely climb twenty stairs.

At the end of the second year, I was angry and depressed.

On my birthday, with my husband on his way to pick up my cake, I went to my room, closed the door and fell on the bed crying.

When I had spent all of the tears and didn't have an ounce of energy left, I heard a voice inside my head. It wasn't the same kind of voice that I hear when I'm talking to myself or remembering what someone said. In fact, it was a male voice.

"Slow down," it said.

"I have slowed down," I answered, still wondering where this voice was coming from. I wondered if this was an angel.

"Listen to your body," it said. "Observe the emotions that come from your pain. Make friends with them. Let them tell you what they want and need. Breathe into them."

Make friends with emotions that come from pain? I had no idea what that meant. I was raised to "turn the other cheek." That meant to ignore what didn't feel good. Even thinking about "them" as being able to speak to me seemed crazy. But I had nothing to lose.

I sat upright in bed, leaned my head against the wall and closed my eyes. Once I felt relaxed, a picture of a gray cloud hanging in space drifted into my mind's eye. I swallowed hard and said, "Hi, depression, I know you're there."

The depression didn't say anything back, but I persisted. "I'm sorry you hurt."

The depression still didn't say anything, but I felt my body relax and let go of tension I wasn't even aware was there. New energy seemed to flow into my body.

The next day when I took time to converse with my depression, a memory emerged. At age nine, when I had rheumatic fever, I was cut off from the outside world. "Contagious: Do Not Enter," was posted on my bedroom door. It was another time when my muscles ached, and I felt weak. I slept off and on for nine months. When I finally recovered, no one mentioned my illness.

"I'm sorry you had to stay in bed, locked in your room," I said to my nine-year-old past self. Tears rushed down my face and landed on my chest. Again, new energy rushed into my body.

The depression I felt with chronic fatigue was

very similar to the depression I felt as a child with rheumatic fever. With both, I'd struggled to get through the pain, but never allowed myself to feel the pain. At age nine, I didn't know how to express my losses. At age forty-eight, I was beginning to understand.

Making friends with my emotions meant noticing the losses, past and present, feeling them, and learning from them.

Now I call that voice I hear my Inner Wisdom. It is a quieter voice than it was when I was ill, but it is still very present in my daily life. As I let go of what I already know and move into the awareness that comes from listening to my so-called bad feelings, a shift occurs. This shift leads me to a peaceful place inside of myself that feeds my soul. It moves me from stress to serenity.

♥ *Judith Fraser, MFT*

The New (Unstressed) You!

Stress can turn you into someone you're not meant to be. You're not meant to be an irritable, short-tempered person in pain and at risk of serious illness—that's not your True Self. If you believe that your life has a purpose, then it's imperative that you develop your True Self to fulfill that purpose. Stress pulls you away from that process.

No matter what your stress style—whether you're an adrenaline junkie or hate to have your routine changed—it can be hard to know when and where to get help for stress. But once you've found the path to peace, you'll see that things will start to change. For example, you'll:

- Feel more energetic and full of life. Stress zaps you of energy, making you feel lethargic and irritable. Beating stress will help you get that energy back and boost your mood.
- Stay healthier. Stress can cause or worsen health problems ranging from headaches to heart disease.
- Enjoy your life more. You'll look forward to every day more when you're feeling calm and relaxed.
- Be a positive influence on those around you. When others see how calm and de-stressed you

are, you may inspire them to want the same for themselves.

Yes, you're on your way to a healthier and more fulfilling life and to becoming your True Self. According to a Chinese proverb, "Tension is who you think you should be. Relaxation is who you are."

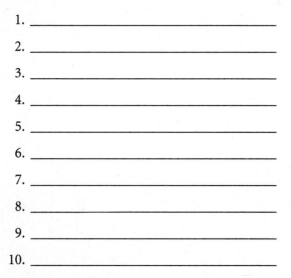

Think about . . .
positive changes in my life

Here are the positive changes I'm looking forward to now that I'm on my way to being less stressed:

1. _____

2. _____

3. _____

4. _____

5. _____

6. _____

7. _____

8. _____

9. _____

10. _____

Don't just eliminate bad habits. Let the positive developments you list above pull you toward a less stressed and more satisfying life. Remember why you're going to the trouble to make lasting changes in your life. The more you focus on these new,

healthier habits and lifestyle changes, the more the
process will take on a life of its own—and the less
work it will take to continue to make your life less
stressful and more satisfying.

Resources

Organizations

Dietitians of Canada provides nutrition information, FAQs, tips on healthy eating and helps consumers find dietitians in their local area. Contact them at:

480 University Avenue, Suite 604, Toronto, ON M5G 1V2
416-596-0857, *www.dietitians.ca*

National Center for Post-Traumatic Stress Disorder:
www.ncptsd.va.gov/

Canadian Mental Health Association:
www.cmha.ca/english/coping_with_stress/

Canadian Traumatic Stress Network:
www.ctsn-rcst.ca

Books

- Beattie, Melody. *Codependent No More: How to Stop Controlling Others and Start Caring for Yourself.* Culver City, MN: Hazelden Publishing & Educational Services, 1996.
- Rubin, Manning. *60 Ways to Relieve Stress in 60 Seconds.* New York City, NY: Workman Publishing, 1993.
- Gladstar, Rosemary. *Herbs for Reducing Stress & Anxiety.* U.S.A.: Storey Publishing, 1999.
- Bodian, Stephan. *Meditations for Dummies.* Foster City, CA: For Dummies, 1999.
- Csikszentmihalyi, Mihaly. *Finding Flow: The Psychology of Engagement with Everyday Life.* New York: Basic Books, 1998.
- Godwin, Leslie. *From Burned Out to Fired Up: A Woman's Guide to Rekindling the Passion and Meaning in Work and Life.* Deerfield Beach, FL: Health Communications, Inc., 2004 *www.LeslieGodwin.com*
- St. James, Elaine. *Living the Simple Life: A Guide to Scaling Down and Enjoying More.* New York: Hyperion Books, 1998.

Who Is Jack Canfield, Cocreator of
Chicken Soup for the Soul®?

Jack Canfield is one of America's leading experts in the development of human potential and personal effectiveness. He is both a dynamic, entertaining speaker and a highly sought-after trainer. Jack has a wonderful ability to inform and inspire audiences toward increased levels of self-esteem and peak performance. He has coauthored numerous books, including *Dare to Win, The Aladdin Factor, 100 Ways to Build Self-Concept in the Classroom, Heart at Work,* and *The Power of Focus.* His latest book is *The Success Principles.*
www.jackcanfield.com

Who Is Mark Victor Hansen, Cocreator of
Chicken Soup for the Soul®?

In the area of human potential, no one is more respected than **Mark Victor Hansen**. For more than thirty years, Mark has focused solely on helping people from all walks of life reshape their personal vision of what's possible. His powerful messages of possibility, opportunity and action have created powerful change in thousands of organizations and millions of individuals nationwide. He is a prolific writer of bestselling books such as *The One Minute Millionaire, The Power of Focus, The Aladdin Factor* and *Dare to Win.*
www.markvictorhansen.com

Who Is Leslie Godwin, MFCC?

Leslie Godwin is a career and life-transition coach specializing in helping physically, emotionally and spiritually exhausted professionals feel revitalized with a fresh viewpoint on their career goals. She is the author of *From Burned Out to Fired Up: A Woman's Guide to Rekindling the Passion and Meaning in Work and Life* (Published by Health Communications, Inc.).

Leslie has been a resource for the *Wall Street Journal, Businessweek.com, Fortune, USAToday.com,* CNN, the Lifetime television network, *Ladies Home Journal, Entrepreneur Magazine, Los Angeles Times, Los Angeles Daily News, www.DrLaura.com,* and other print and online media. She lives in Calabasas, California with her husband, Bob, their son, Tristan, and their Harlequin Great Dane, Savannah.
www.lesliegodwin.com

Who Is Linda Formichelli?

Linda Formichelli writes on health, self-help and other topics for *Family Circle, USA Weekend, Fitness, Writer's Digest, Oxygen* and other magazines. She's the coauthor of several books, including *The Renegade Writer: A Totally Unconventional Guide to Freelance Writing Success,* which helps writers break into magazine writing and make more money by breaking the rules. Linda lives in Concord, New Hampshire, with her writer husband and two cats.
www.lindaformichelli.com

Contributors

Isabel Bearman Bucher is unto herself first, where all things must begin. She's a wife, mother of two grown daughters, sister and friend. After retiring from twenty years of teaching elementary school, she was able to begin her honeymoon with life. She and Robert travel the world doing home exchanges; she writes, exercises, hikes and wonders sometimes where the years have all gone. She's working on her first work of fiction, *Tafoya's Laundromat,* set in 1969 Taos, New Mexico.

Judith Morton Fraser, MFT, is a marriage-family therapist from Los Angeles. Her personal experience with a life-altering illness inspired Judith to write *What's So Good About Bad Feelings,* a self-help book that encourages others to learn from life's difficulties.

Cynthia Hinkle is the author of the 2005 Christmas Arch® Book *Star of Wonder* and a contributing author in *God Answers Prayers—Military Edition.* She lives with son Peter, daughter Jessica, research scientist Andrew Hinkle and two cats in southwest Ohio. Her eldest son, Michael, is an OSU graduate in Industrial Design.

Abha Iyengar has contributed to *Knit Lit Too; Chicken Soup for the Healthy Soul—Menopause; Science, Technology and Development* and other print anthologies. She is a Kota Press Poetry Anthology Contest winner. Her work has appeared in *Raven Chronicles, Gowanus Books, Tattoo Highway, riverbabble, Moondance* and *Writers Against War,* among other publications.

Patricia Jones lived in New York City with her daughter. Her work has appeared in *Ms., Essence, Family Circle, Woman's Day* and the *New York Times.* Patrica wrote three novels, *Passing, Red on a Rose* and her final novel, *The Color of Family.*

Dolores Kozielski is a certified feng shui practitioner, trained in Kabbalah, Qigong, t'ai chi, meditational Chinese brush stroke and the art of iconography. She is a professional author and an award-winning poet, published with major publishing houses including HarperCollins and Scholastic. Dolores may be reached at *www.FengShuiWrite.com.*

Jennifer Lawler is the author of more than twenty books, including her popular *Dojo Wisdom* series (Penguin Compass). She writes about martial arts, parenting and self-help for major consumer magazines. Her Web site is *www.jenniferlawler.com.* She lives in the Midwest with her daughter, Jessica, and two rambunctious dogs.

Larisa Migachyov obtained her Master's Degree in biomechanical engineering from Standford University, and spent several years working in Silicon Valley. She now owns a small math tutoring practice. Her hobbies include piano playing, downhill skiing, and versification.

Sallie A. Rodman has a Certificate in Professional Writing from California State University, Long Beach. Her works have appeared in many magazines, newspapers, *Chicken Soup* anthologies and the *Chocolate for Women* series. She is currently working on a book about her life with panic attacks. She has three grown children who live around the globe. Sallie lives in Los Alamitos, California, with a husband, a cat and a dog. So far, they are not published. Contact her at *sa.rodman@verizon.net.*

Michael Jordan Segal, MSW, is a social worker, author, husband, father and inspirational speaker. His miraculous comeback story was first published in *Chicken Soup for the Christian Family Soul.* Since then he has had many stories published in anthologies, magazines and newspapers. To contact Mike, please visit *www.InspirationByMike.com* or call Sterling International Speakers Bureau at 1-877-226-1003.

Sarah Skilton lives in Los Angeles with her husband/college sweetheart, Joe. Her work has appeared in local and national magazines, DVDs and audio CDs. She loves to travel, occasionally knits scarves and is hard at work on her first novel. For all things Sarah, visit: *www.sarahskilton.com*

Shirley Warren describes her writing as the best excuse she can find for avoiding housework. Her works are based on her desire to find inspiration in ordinary day-to-day experiences. She resides in Massachusetts with her husband and son, where they choose to live happily ever after one day at a time.

Winnie Yu is the coauthor of three books, including *What to Do When the Doctor Says It's Early-Stage Alzheimer's* (Fair Winds Press, 2005). Her work has appeared in several national magazines, including *Woman's Day, Redbook, Weight Watchers, Fitness* and *Parents.* She lives in upstate New York with her husband, Jeff, and two daughters.

Permissions

Get the perfect blend of information and inspiration.

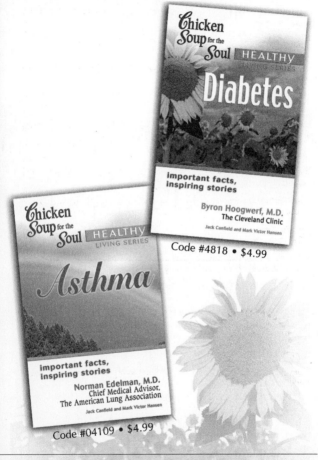

Also Available

Chicken Soup African American Soul
Chicken Soup Body and Soul
Chicken Soup Bride's Soul
Chicken Soup Caregiver's Soul
Chicken Soup Cat and Dog Lover's Soul
Chicken Soup Christian Family Soul
Chicken Soup Christian Soul
Chicken Soup College Soul
Chicken Soup Country Soul
Chicken Soup Couple's Soul
Chicken Soup Expectant Mother's Soul
Chicken Soup Father's Soul
Chicken Soup Fisherman's Soul
Chicken Soup Girlfriend's Soul
Chicken Soup Golden Soul
Chicken Soup Golfer's Soul, Vol. I, II
Chicken Soup Horse Lover's Soul
Chicken Soup Inspire a Woman's Soul
Chicken Soup Kid's Soul
Chicken Soup Mother's Soul, Vol. I, II
Chicken Soup Nature Lover's Soul
Chicken Soup Parent's Soul
Chicken Soup Pet Lover's Soul
Chicken Soup Preteen Soul, Vol. I, II
Chicken Soup Single's Soul
Chicken Soup Soul, Vol. I-VI
Chicken Soup at Work
Chicken Soup Sports Fan's Soul
Chicken Soup Teenage Soul, Vol. I-IV
Chicken Soup Woman's Soul, Vol. I, II
